Advancing Health Literacy

Christina Zarcadoolas
Andrew F. Pleasant
David S. Greer

Advancing Health Literacy

A Framework for Understanding and Action

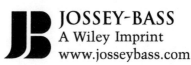

JOSSEY-BASS
A Wiley Imprint
www.josseybass.com

Published by Jossey-Bass
A Wiley Imprint
989 Market Street, San Francisco, CA 94103-1741   www.josseybass.com

Jossey-Bass books and products are available through most bookstores. To contact Jossey-Bass directly call our Customer Care Department within the U.S. at 800-956-7739, outside the U.S. at 317-572-3986, or fax 317-572-4002.

Jossey-Bass also publishes its books in a variety of electronic formats. Some content that appears in print may not be available in electronic books.

Library of Congress Cataloging-in-Publication Data

Zarcadoolas, Christina, 1948–
    Advancing health literacy : a framework for understanding and action / Christina Zarcadoolas, Andrew F. Pleasant, David S. Greer.
        p. ; cm.
    Includes bibliographical references and index.
    ISBN-13: 978-0-7879-8433-5 (pbk.)
    ISBN-10: 0-7879-8433-7 (pbk.)
    1. Health education.   2. Patient education.   3. Literacy.   I. Pleasant, Andrew F., 1962–   II. Greer, David S.   III. Title.
    [DNLM: 1. Health Education. 2. Educational Status. WA 590 Z36a 2006]
    RA440.5.Z37 2006
    613—dc22   2006013528

Printed in the United States of America
FIRST EDITION
PB Printing   10 9 8 7 6 5 4 3 2 1

Contents

List of Tables, Figures, and Exhibits

Tables

Figures

Exhibits

Preface

A silent killer maneuvers just below the surface of almost all the health issues that will lead to death and disease in the 21st century. The U.S. population faces well-recognized health risks, including chronic diseases, environmental degradation, and natural and man-made disasters, but the silent killer is less diagnosed and remains essentially untreated. The silent killer is low health literacy: the reality that almost half of adults in the United States, over 90 million people, struggle to find, understand, and correctly use health information.

For example, people with low or inadequate health literacy find it difficult, if not impossible, to accurately read instructions for taking medications, understand their health plan restrictions, understand and act on public health warnings, or accurately read evacuation plans and other emergency information. Major health policy reports such as *Healthy People 2010* strongly link poor education, low literacy, poor health, and early death in the United States and around the rest of the world. Disasters such as the terrorist attacks on September 11, 2001, and Hurricane Katrina in 2005 have tragically demonstrated that poor communication can be deadly. Low health literacy is one of the most unheralded yet critical threats to public health.

This book outlines a new model of health literacy, applies the model to the analysis of public health messages in a series of case studies, and presents best-practice guidelines for communicating health messages. The model addresses skills and abilities that people use to understand and act on health information and demonstrates how health professionals can use these insights to communicate more effectively and advance health literacy. In this book, we take an inclusive view of literacy by defining it as a rich and varied range of skills and abilities: the repertoire of resources a person or group of people have, or can develop, to understand and act on information.

The Goal of This Book

Our goal is to answer the following question: How can this model of health literacy and the literacy principles it outlines improve the daily performance of health professionals and health programs in their efforts to advance individual and public health literacy?

We explore and answer a number of questions: What are the goals of communicating with the public about health? How are health issues currently being communicated? Is the language used easy to read, listen to, and understand? What core concepts and vocabulary are essential? If we acknowledge that people will understand messages at different levels, are the messages constructed so that this can actually occur? Is the public able to absorb and use health information in a meaningful way? Does health communication advance the public's understanding of health, science, and technology?

We define *health literacy* as the ability to understand, evaluate, and act on spoken, written, and visual health information to reduce risk and live a healthier life. It is more than the ability to read health information. Health literacy is made up of a broad range of skills—some complex, some mundane—that allow people to make health care decisions and to advocate for themselves, their family, and their community. Adequate health literacy is one path to improved health and quality of life.

Consequences of Low Health Literacy

The consequences of low health literacy include poorer health outcomes, increased risk in emergency situations, lack of social empowerment and self-efficacy, and the financial costs associated with a less healthy population. There are other consequences, including an increased burden on health care providers when they treat people who do not adhere to medical treatments and preventive measures because of their lack of understanding. Low health literacy also results in the overuse or misuse of the health care system, which drives up costs. Consider these examples of the results of low health literacy:

• The American Medical Association's (AMA) health literacy initiative has demonstrated that many patients cannot read and understand directions on their prescription bottles.

• It is estimated that low reading level and low health literacy may be responsible for up to $69 billion in additional health expenditures in the United States (Institute of Medicine, 2003). This reflects improper understanding of medical regimens such as improper use of prescription and over-the-counter medications, poor understanding of medical treatment options, and poor understanding of risk avoidance and health prevention.

• Many chronic diseases, such as diabetes, heart disease, and high blood pressure, go undiagnosed or unsuccessfully treated.

• There is poor understanding of the role of health literacy in dealing with large-scale natural disasters, as well as newly emergent risks such as bioterrorism.

• There is poor understanding of the role of health literacy among health experts and public health officials.

• Effective communication between the public and professionals about health and environmental health risks in a community is often missing, especially in the presence of scientific uncertainty.

- Positive health behavior change is less likely when people do not have information about the environment, science, disease processes, and preventive measures that they can understand.
- Timely response to emergency situations and disasters is less possible when people do not have information they can understand and executable directions to guarantee their safety.
- People with low income, low educational level, and low literacy level and members of racial and ethnic minority groups often have higher illness and mortality rates.

Health promotion and education efforts urgently need to identify relevant characteristics of individuals and groups in order to design effective health messages and campaigns. The success of health promotion depends on bridging the content of health promotion to individuals. Health literacy skills make that possible.

What Does Hard-to-Understand Health Information Look Like?

Within the world of medicine and health care, complex information is so commonplace that it is often very difficult for professionals to recognize the barriers this information presents to the public. If the gap between message and audience were found only rarely or only in the elite media, there would be less cause for concern. Unfortunately, complexity is far more ubiquitous. For instance, following the 2001 terrorist attacks on the United States and the later anthrax incidents, the health web site WebMD presented the following explanation of anthrax that poses many barriers for people with low health literacy:

What Is Anthrax?

For thousands of years, anthrax—an animal disease—has been around. The bacterium is called *Bacillus anthracis*, which can "seed" itself and produce long-lasting spores.

These spores can stay in the environment a long time. The bacterium produces toxins that cause three types of anthrax. In cases of exposure, one has come in contact with a small amount of bacteria, but enough to cause the disease. Anthrax is not contagious.

This communication raises a number of questions:

- Does the public:

  Have the reading ability to understand *bacterium* and *Bacillus anthracis*?

  Have a working concept of what a spore is? Is it important that they have this knowledge?

  Have the ability to use this information to help judge their personal risk and take appropriate actions?

If the answers are no, how do we respond?

While the twentieth century saw a dramatic decrease in death from communicable diseases, primarily thanks to antimicrobials and improved hygiene, the 21st century will likely see an increase in death and disability from chronic conditions, including heart disease and cancer, as well as mental health conditions and other illnesses related to lifestyle and behavior (Institute for the Future, 2003). People who have a broad range of literacy skills can take part in the personal and public dialogue on issues that are important to their lives and well-being as well as those of others.

The Growing Complexity of Medicine and Health

There is a growing movement to better understand how experts communicate with the general public and what that public needs to understand about often complex and changing science and health information. This movement toward creating a more literate public is partially driven by the apparent disconnect between

knowledge, science, and technology and what the public understands of those issues.

In genomics, scientists tell us that the identification of the complete structure of human DNA will enable the development of new
treatments for some of our most perplexing health problems. How
likely is it that the general public can understand this dramatic
breakthrough and use it effectively? What would they need to
understand to develop informed public judgment about stem cell
research or cloning, or to assess the differences between human
reproductive cloning and nuclear transplantation? As medical science and technology advance at an accelerated pace, there is danger that individuals and the public will fail to master critical
knowledge, to the detriment of their health and well-being.

What You Will Find in This Book

In Chapter 1 we define health literacy and use examples of complex, high-barrier messages and easy-to-understand, low-barrier messages to clarify the problem. We discuss the changing demographics
of the country and the implications for public health officials and
other health providers.

We place the discussion of health literacy in a historical context
in Chapter 2, looking at the movement from public health education in the early 1900s, to the current models of the health consumer and shared decision making.

In Chapter 3 we redefine health literacy, broadening the definition to include four critical domains: fundamental, scientific, civic,
and cultural literacy.

In Chapter 4 we present basic language and reading theory and
discuss how language and reading work. We discuss models from linguistics, communications, and social marketing to analyze a range
of health communications.

In Chapter 5 we discuss how the media work in setting the
agenda, framing, and disseminating health information. We explain

the function and meaning of several models of mass communication, including social marketing.

In Chapter 6 we discuss the newest mass communication medium, the internet, which growing numbers of people are using to access health information. We discuss issues of access, understandability, and trust that arise in that communication context.

Chapters 7 through 13 present a series of case studies of actual health communications. Each case highlights a different domain discussed in our health literacy model: prenatal health education, genomics, smoking cessation, anthrax, HIV/AIDS, diabetes, and breast cancer.

In Chapter 14, we present best-practice guidelines for writing and designing linguistically and culturally appropriate health information using health literacy principles discussed in the book.

Health and health literacy are powerfully linked, and every health communication can be an opportunity to foster both. Health literacy is now recognized as a major public health issue. The purpose of this book is to provide health professionals, communicators, and students with the insights and the tools they will need to communicate effectively in a rapidly evolving and increasingly complex environment.

Acknowledgments

We thank the following people who assisted along the way: our students Andrea Balazs, Marian Thorpe, and Nathan James and our colleagues and collaborators Wei Ying Wong; Polly Reynolds; Sabrina Kurtz-Rossi, Sally Waldron, and Judy Titzel of World Education; Lisa Bernstein at the What to Expect Foundation; and Kibbe Conti, who introduced us to the Four Winds Nutrition Model. A National Library of Medicine publication grant made this work's start a possibility, and we thank the library. There would be no final product without the dedication and patience given to us by Patricia Caton. We also acknowledge the support of Andy Pasternack and everyone else at Jossey-Bass who worked on this book.

The Authors

Christina Zarcadoolas is a sociolinguist who has worked for over 30 years on people's use of spoken and written language. She focuses on how various publics understand health and environmental issues. She began her work as a teacher of the deaf in Rhode Island and New York City. The specific reading challenges of deaf people as well as their unique fluency with visual language served as a major cornerstone for her studies of language in use. Through the study of patient-physician communication in the 1980s and public understanding of environmental issues in the 1990s, she has become nationally known for her work on health and environmental literacy. Her research focuses on analyzing and closing the gaps between expert knowledge and public understanding of health and environmental issues. She was on the faculty at Brown University's Center for Environmental Studies for 15 years, where she designed and taught courses on public perception of the environment and environmental communication and worked with numerous federal, state, and community-based organizations to solve communication problems. She is on the faculty of Mount Sinai School of Medicine in the Department of Community and Preventive Medicine. She is currently working on applying health literacy principles in the area of emergency preparedness. Zarcadoolas received her Ph.D. from Brown University.

Andrew Pleasant works both internationally and within the United States on issues of health literacy; the communication of science, health, and environmental issues; and how individuals and communities can create positive change in order to protect and improve human health and the quality of natural and built environments. Pleasant is an assistant professor in the Department of Human Ecology and the Department of Family and Community Health Sciences at Rutgers, the State University of New Jersey. Prior to earning a master's degree in environmental studies from Brown University and a Ph.D. in communication from Cornell University, he worked as a photojournalist, journalist, and editor at daily newspapers in the United States.

David S. Greer joined the administration and faculty of the new medical school at Brown University in 1974. He founded and chaired the Department of Family Medicine, the Department of Community Health, and the Gerontology Center at Brown University in Providence, Rhode Island. In 1981, he was appointed dean of medicine at Brown and remained in that position until 1992.

Greer has been a family doctor, researcher, medical school leader, community leader, and mentor to countless health professionals for many decades. During the 1960s and 1970s, he founded the first hospital-connected public housing facility for the physically impaired in the nation based in Fall River, Massachusetts. His geriatric career began with his interest in housing and community support, which led to federal funding for Highland Heights Apartments. This was a prototype of the now-ubiquitous assisted living facilities in the United States.

Greer's honors and awards include an honorary doctor of humane letters from Southeastern Massachusetts University, the Distinguished Service Award from the University of Chicago Medical Alumni Association, and the Outstanding Citizen Award from the Jewish Veterans Auxiliary. Greer received his B.S. from the University of Notre Dame and M.D. from the University of Chicago. He was a founding director of International Physicians for the Prevention of Nuclear War, which won the Nobel Peace Prize in 1985.

Advancing Health Literacy

1

Health Literacy
Why Is It a Public Health Issue?

More than half the adults in the United States find it difficult, if not impossible, to understand their health plan coverage, read instructions for taking medications and drug interactions, or understand and act on public health warnings. These tasks are a function of health literacy, which we can begin defining as a person's ability to find, understand, and act on health information. While we will expand and elaborate on this definition throughout this book and present a new framework for understanding health literacy, this chapter establishes the fundamentals of why health literacy is a major public health issue that can and should be addressed by health professionals in many fields. (A number of important government and academic initiatives are now focused on health literacy: Ad Hoc Committee on Health Literacy, 1999; U.S. Department of Health and Human Services, 2000; Schwartzberg, VanGeest, & Wang, 2005; Partnership for Clear Health Communication, 2003; Nielsen-Bohlman, Panzer, & Kindig, 2004.)

Low health literacy contributes to a number of difficulties:

- Improper use of medications

- Inappropriate use or no use of health services

- Poor self-management of chronic conditions

- Inadequate response in emergency situations

- Poor health outcomes

- Lack of self-efficacy and self-esteem

- Financial drain on individuals and society

- Social inequity

The following are three examples of the dire consequences of the inability to successfully educate people about better health prevention and disease management in the United States:

- *Type 2 diabetes.* Diabetes is the seventh leading cause of death in the United States, directly affecting 6.2 percent of the population (17 million people). The disease disproportionately affects minority populations. Non-Latino blacks, Latino Americans, American Indians, and Alaska Natives all have a higher prevalence of diabetes than non-Latino whites. American Indians and Alaska Natives have the highest prevalence of diabetes (15.1 percent) of any racial/ethnic group studied (National Diabetes Information Clearinghouse, 2002). Type 2 diabetes is largely a lifestyle illness.
- *HIV/AIDS.* The rate of HIV infection has hovered at over 40,000 new cases per year since 1998. The rate of decline has slowed significantly, from 13 percent in 1997 to 3 percent in 1999. Minority groups disproportionately represent the highest rates of new infections. Blacks represent 12 percent of the general population yet make up 54 percent of new infections. Women between the ages of 13 and 24, especially women of color, make up 47 percent of HIV cases. There has been a resurgence of cases in young men who have sex with men, a group that previously showed dramatic declines in infection rates associated with intense education (Centers for Disease Control and Prevention, 2001).
- *Maternal and newborn health.* Roughly 4 million infants are born in the United States each year. Among developed countries,

the United States is ranked 25th in infant mortality (National Center for Health Statistics, 2001) and 21st in maternal mortality (World Health Organization, United Nations Population Fund, United Nations Children's Fund, & World Bank, 1999). While the infant mortality rate dropped more than 22 percent in the United States between 1991 and 2000 (6.9 percent of live births), black infants are more than twice as likely to die as white infants, and Hispanic women are three to four times as likely to die in childbirth in the United States (Division of Reproductive Health, n.d.). Preterm births occur in 9.7 percent of all U.S. births, yet the rate for blacks is double that of whites and the rate is 25 percent higher for Hispanics than for whites (Reagan & Salsberry, 2004). The proportion of all babies born with low birth weight in the United States between 1991 and 2000 increased 7 percent (March of Dimes, 2003). Financial cost is also embedded in these statistics. The average cost of caring for the tiniest newborns now exceeds $200,000, according to researchers (Preidt, 2005).

The role of women's health literacy is important in these sobering statistics. For example, while it is believed that up to 70 percent of birth defects of the brain and spinal cord may be prevented if women take 4 milligrams (4,000 micrograms) of folic acid daily prior to and during early weeks of pregnancy, in 2002 only 31 percent of nonpregnant women surveyed said that they were taking a daily multivitamin containing folic acid. And those least likely to be consuming folic acid included women ages 18 to 24, women who had not attended college, and women with annual household incomes under $25,000 (March of Dimes, 2003).

The greater prevalence of chronic disease, technological and scientific revolutions, and globalization, including both the quicker spread of communicable diseases and the threats of bioterrorism, all set the stage for substantive changes in what public health means and how to attain it for the largest number of citizens (Institute of Medicine, 2003). The terrorist attacks on the United States of

September 11, 2001, demonstrated both weaknesses and strengths in the public health system (Institute of Medicine, 2003). Much criticism points beyond infrastructure problems and toward communication problems—for example, federal, state, and local officials' inadequacies in communicating with one another and the general public (Connolly, 2001). The Institute of Medicine (2003) summed up this critical need: "Therefore, the committee recommends that all partners within the public health system place special emphasis on communication as a critical core competency of public health practice. Government public health agencies at all levels should use existing and emerging tools (including information technologies) for effective management of public health information and for internal and external communication. To be effective, such communication must be culturally appropriate and suitable to the literacy levels of the individuals in the communities they serve" (p. 125).

As we will discuss next, health literacy refers to more than reading and writing. It refers as well to the powerful skills that make it possible for people to talk about, know, and organize health information.

Definitions of Key Terms

Often the terms *health communication*, *health promotion*, and *health education* are used interchangeably. Because the discussion throughout this book uses all of these terms, we will use the following definitions, based on the 1998 WHO Health Promotion Glossary, greatly influenced by the Ottawa Charter for Health Promotion and the Jakarta Declaration of 1997 (Nutbeam, 1998).

Health promotion is the "process of enabling people to increase control over and to improve their health" (World Health Organization, 1998, p. 11). The mission of public health is actualized through health promotion and disease prevention. Health promotion relies on health education and health communication, as well as systems and policies that advance the public's health status.

Health education is the full range of activities that involve communicating health information to people. It attempts to address the gap between what we know about health and what people actually practice (Glanz & Rudd, 1990; Griffiths, 1972). Health education can take place anywhere: in the home or community, schools and health care settings, work sites, and the consumer marketplace (Glanz & Rudd, 1990).

Health communication is the use of human and mass or multimedia and other communication skills and technologies to educate or inform an individual or public about a health issue and to keep that issue on the public agenda. Study after study has concluded that most consumers want more and better health information. A key objective is to construct linguistically, culturally appropriate, and innovative communications using the public health system and to have better patient-provider encounters.

Social marketing is the merging of traditional marketing and advertising strategies to persuade people to act in specific ways on social issues such as health and the environment (Andreason, 1995; McKenzie-Mohr & Smith, 1999). Social marketing focuses on designing and evaluating messages and campaigns through careful audience analysis, segmentation, identification of target audiences (market segmentation), understanding those audiences, and ultimately tailoring communications for a desired effect. Instead of starting with what an audience does not know and needs to know, the social marketer begins with knowing what people do and do not do, and why. The goal is behavior change.

Consumer decision making involves the active cognitive and emotional roles individuals play in attending to, evaluating, and acting on health information. Ever more frequently, health consumers are required to become more active coparticipants in their health and health care. Some examples are making medical treatment decisions, choosing health plans, or making decisions about lifestyle changes.

Health literacy is the wide range of skills and competencies that people develop to seek out, comprehend, evaluate, and use health information and concepts to make informed choices, reduce health risks, and increase quality of life. (We elaborate on this definition in Chapter 3.)

Medical Information

If the quantity of health information were the litmus test for a health-literate population, there would not be a health problem in the United States. Information about health in the United States is ubiquitous. As a society, we are awash with health messages—most too complicated, many often misleading. We receive health information from many sources: doctors, family and friends, television, newspapers, magazines, and the internet. Direct-to-consumer marketing by the pharmaceutical industry as well as online purchase of medications has created a climate in which the consumer is more and more able to ask for and receive commercially marketed products (David & Greer, 2001; Kaphingst, Rudd, DeJong, & Daltroy, 2004a).

Complexity of Health Information and Materials

Health education and promotion are critical for reaching and empowering the public in general and vulnerable people in particular. And yet much health education and promotion material in print and on the internet is written at the tenth-grade reading level or higher, far out of the reach of the average patient or consumer (Doak, Doak, & Root, 1996; Williams et al., 1995; Zarcadoolas, Ahern, & Blanco, 1997). The most easily identifiable complexity comes in the sentences and words we use. For example, the following health information texts are at the 12th- to 15th-grade level:

Navigating the Health Care System: Medicaid

The law cited below [not included here] requires that all conditions of eligibility must be verified at each redetermination of eligibility unless the verification is pending from a third party and the recipient has cooperated in obtaining the verification. Since you have not provided the necessary verification or you have failed to cooperate in obtaining verification from a third party, your cash and/or medical assistance must be stopped.

This is very hard to read for several reasons:

- High-level vocabulary (*cited*, *eligibility*, *redetermination*, and *verification*, for example)

- Long and complex sentences

- Passive versus active sentences ("the recipient has co-operated in obtaining . . .")

Unfortunately, it is rare that only the vocabulary or sentences are complex. The following example is from a fact sheet on colorectal cancer from the American Cancer Society (2006) titled "What Are the Risk Factors for Colorectal Cancer?" Here, two important ingredients add to the complexity: the reader needs to know some basics about risk and risk factors and also needs to have skill in numeracy to understand personal risk.

A *risk factor* is anything that increases your chance of getting a disease such as cancer. Different cancers have different risk factors. For example, unprotected exposure to strong sunlight is a risk factor for skin cancer, and smoking is a risk factor for cancers of the lungs, larynx, mouth, throat, esophagus, kidneys, bladder, colon, and several other organs. Researchers have identified several risk factors that increase a person's chance of developing colorectal polyps or colorectal cancer.

A *family history of colorectal cancer:* If you have a first-degree relative (parent, sibling, or offspring) who has had colorectal cancer, your risk for developing this disease is increased. People who have two or more close relatives with colorectal cancer make up about 20 percent of all people with colorectal cancer. The risk increases even further if the relatives are affected before the age of 60. About 5 percent to 10 percent of patients with colorectal cancer have an inherited genetic abnormality that causes the cancer. One abnormality is called *familial adenomatous polyposis (FAP)* and a second is called *hereditary nonpolyposis colorectal cancer (HNPCC)*, also known as Lynch syndrome. These abnormalities are described later in this document. No other clearly identified genetic abnormalities have been described at this time.

And when complex messages convey complex issues, low-literate people are placed in a kind of triple jeopardy: they cannot understand the information, they cannot judge the trustworthiness of the information, and they are forced to rely on information that is difficult to understand and may be unreliable (for example, a community rumor, a sensationalist media broadcast, or scare tactics of special interests groups.)

Consider the following example of a communication about BSE from a U.S. Department of Agriculture (2005) press release:

Since the USDA enhanced surveillance program for BSE [bovine spongiform encephalopathy] began in June 2004, more than 375,000 animals from the targeted cattle population have been tested for BSE using a rapid test. Three of these animals tested inconclusive and were subsequently subjected to immunohistochemistry, or IHC, testing. The IHC is an internationally recognized confirmatory test for BSE. All three inconclusive samples tested negative using IHC.

Earlier this week, USDA's Office of the Inspector General (OIG), which has been partnering with the Animal and Plant Health Inspection Service, the Food Safety and Inspection Service, and the Agricultural Research Service by impartially reviewing BSE-related activities and making recommendations for improvement, recommended that all three of these samples be subjected to a second internationally recognized confirmatory test, the OIE-recognized SAF immunoblot test, often referred to as the Western blot test. We received final results a short time ago. Of the three samples, two were negative, but the third came back reactive.

Because of the conflicting results on the IHC and Western blot tests, a sample from this animal will be sent to the OIE-recognized reference laboratory for BSE in Weybridge, England. USDA will also be conducting further testing, which will take several days to complete.

Regardless of the outcome, it is critical to note that USDA has in place a sound system of interlocking safeguards to protect human and animal health from BSE—including, most significantly, a ban on specified risk materials from the human food supply. In the case of this animal, it was a non-ambulatory (downer) animal and as such was banned from the food supply. It was processed at a facility that handles only animals unsuitable for human consumption, and the carcass was incinerated.

This press release combines all of the sins of failed health communication, with the result that it is incomprehensible to the vast majority of the U.S. population. It contains high-level language and obscure scientific terms that unnecessarily complicate the message. Buried at the end, implied, but never directly stated, is the reassurance the public needs: "don't worry—the government is able to safeguard your supply of meat—you won't be poisoned by sick cows." Of course, health communicators must be careful to stick to the known facts rather than to simply attempt to persuade the public that all is well when it is either not well or unknown. The early British government response to BSE in which John Gummer, then the secretary of state for the environment, created a photo opportunity by stuffing a hamburger into his little daughter's mouth is now a notorious example of an ill-conceived strategy to calm the public when scientific uncertainty about the threat remained high. The outcome of efforts that are not based in honest communication strategies can often be increased distrust and outrage (Jasanoff, 1997).

Providing Information in Languages Other Than English

Perhaps as important as addressing complexity are the lack of availability of easy-to-read and understand materials in languages other than English and the need for health promotion methods that are culturally sensitive.

As indicated by the 1990 Census, 14 percent of the population in the United States speaks a language other than English (31.8 million persons). The main languages spoken are English, Spanish, Chinese, French, German, Tagalog, and Vietnamese.

Regardless of language or culture, one thing that appears to be universal is that people want and need information about their health, especially when they or their family members are ill. Yet often people do not have the answers to their basic questions:

- What is the medical problem, and how is it diagnosed?

- What is the right treatment for me?

- Can I trust the information I am getting?

- What do I have to do to be healthier?

- What are my risk factors for a disease?

- How do I use the health care system effectively?

- How does my medical insurance work?

The Relationship Between Health and Literacy

Low literacy, poor health, and early death are strongly linked in this country and around the world (Clenland & Van Ginniken, 1988; Grosse & Auffrey, 1989; Hohn, 1997; Tresserras, Canela, Alvarez, Sentis, & Salleras, 1992). In the mid-1990s a series of studies clearly linked low literacy level to patient health behaviors. In a study of patients at two urban public hospitals, one in Atlanta and the other in Los Angeles, Williams et al. (1995, p. 1677) assessed the functional health literacy among English-speaking and Spanish-speaking patients. They defined adequate functional health literacy as "the ability to comprehend quantitative information, which may differ from the ability to read a prose passage." They found that up to 33 percent of patients presenting for acute care at these facilities could not adequately understand instructions for a common radiographic procedure written at a fourth-grade level, 24.3 to 58.2 percent of patients did not understand directions to take medication on an empty stomach, and more than 20 percent of patients incorrectly answered questions regarding information on a routinely used appointment slip.

Jolly, Scott, Feied, and Sanford (1993) and Powers (1988) assessed the readability of patient-directed print materials in university hospital emergency departments. They found that a significant number of the patients (more than 50 percent in Powers's study) were not able to read well enough to understand standard discharge information, such as instructions on how to care for wounds or sprains.

Many Americans Are Low-Literate

The National Adult Literacy Survey (NALS) found that approximately 45 percent of the U.S. population (90 million people) has limited literacy (Kirsch, Junegeblut, Jenkins, & Kolstad, 1993). NALS made it possible, for the first time, to construct a detailed picture of the literacy skills of adults in the United States. This study assessed three types of literacy: prose, document, and quantitative. NALS sheds important light on the literacy of older Americans, high consumers of health care, as it indicates that low levels of prose, document, and quantitative literacy are a significant problem for a large portion of the older adult population in the United States (defined as 60 years and older). Among the population age

65 and older, 44 percent tested at the lowest literacy level, level 1 (roughly third to fifth grade level), and 32 percent tested in the second-lowest level, level II. When literacy levels were correlated with physical disabilities, similar results were revealed. For instance, of the population with long-term illness, 70 percent of the affected population performed at the lowest literacy levels.

Do Literacy and Education Go Hand in Hand?

Education level is often used as a proxy for literacy level, presuming the higher the level of education, the higher the literacy level. But as the International Adult Literacy Survey (IALS, 2003) Canadian report indicates, "The connection between educational attainment and literacy levels, while strong, is not exclusive. Many individuals—one third of the population in fact—do not fit the general pattern. But with respect to individuals, their actual literacy may be greater—or less—than their level of education might suggest" (para. 22).

Literacy Problems Among Minorities in the United States

English literacy levels among minorities in the United States are very low, as Table 1.1 shows (levels I and II are fifth-grade level and lower, and level I is below third-grade reading level ability).

What Are the Barriers to Health Literacy?

Among the most recognized barriers to health literacy are the following:

- Complexity of written health information in print and on the web

- Lack of health information in languages other than English

- Lack of cultural appropriateness of health information

- Inaccuracy or incompleteness of information in mass media

- Low-level reading abilities, especially among under-educated, elderly, and some segments of ethnic minority populations

- Lack of empowering content that targets behavior change as well as direct information (social marketing strategies)

Why Is Literacy So Important to Health Promotion?

Literacy is not just about reading and writing. It has powerful individual and social consequences and corollaries (Olson, 1994).

Table 1.1. English Literacy Levels Among Minorities in the United States

Race/Ethnicity	Level I (%)	Level II (%)
Black	46	34
Asian/Pacific Islander	33	23
American Indians	29	37
Other	49	21
Hispanic (Mexicans)	54	25
Hispanic (Cubans)	46	20
Hispanic (Puerto Ricans)	51	28
Hispanic (Central and South Americans)	53	25
Hispanic (other)	31	25

Note: Results of this survey were reported in five levels. Levels I and II were considered to have the lowest literacy.

Source: Kirsch et al. (1993).

Intuitively we understand that people who cannot read (those who are illiterate) or cannot read well (those who are low literate) are handicapped to a great degree in society. Literacy helps us get on in the world; it gives us access and privilege. If you have ever assisted someone who cannot read a train schedule, or overheard a patient asking his wife to read a prescription label for him, or struggled while traveling in a country where another language is mainly spoken, you know in an instant the profound impact literacy has on a person's life.

During the dramatic anthrax events of 2001, a Gallup poll found that individuals with less formal education were more likely to be worried about exposure to anthrax. Forty-four percent of Americans with a high school education or less were worried compared to 21 percent of those with college degree (Jones, 2001). (See the anthrax case study in Chapter 9.) These data suggest that people with higher education levels (and, more likely, higher functional literacy level) may be better able to judge the quality and reliability of information sources and weigh relative risk.

Research from many disciplines contributes to the understanding of literacy. Major contributors include linguists, philosophers, anthropologists, psychologists, cognitive scientists, reading researchers, and educators. Representative of these disciplines are the following: sociolinguistics and discourse analysis (Gumperz, 1982; Hymes, 1974; Labov, 1972, 1994; Stubbs, 1983; Tannen, 1982), social anthropologists (Achard & Kemmer, 2003), text analysts studying narratives (Propp, 1968; van Dijk, 1977), researchers of written and spoken language (Kroll & Vann, 1981; Scribner & Cole, 1981), cognitivists (Luria, 1976; Vygotsky, 1962), and literacy and reading experts (Britton & Graesser, 1996; Olson, 1980; Olson & Torrance, 2001; Orasanu, 1986). Among the central questions that scholars in these fields ask about literacy and language are:

- How do literacy and language influence how we think (cognition)?

- What is the relationship between spoken and written language?

- What happens to our literacy abilities over our lifetime?

- What are the skill differences between less and more literate individuals?

- What kinds of empowerment result from literacy or are a consequence of it?

- How do written, spoken, and visual texts get understood and used?

The consequences of literacy have been closely examined by studying both literate and nonliterate cultures (Goody & Watt, 1968; Havelock, 1973; McLuhan, 1964; Olson, 1977). We know that literacy affects rational thought and the cognitive processing of information (Bruner, 1966; Clanchy, 1979; Greenfield, 1972; Scribner & Cole, 1981; Stock, 1983). Researchers and philosophers over the past 200 years have associated literacy with social progress. Literacy provides a means to create social norms as well as the ability and tacit permission to question them.

Rao and Rao (2002, p. 32) capture this power: "Proper literacy comprises practices and reading and writing which enhance people's control over their lives and their capacity for making rational judgments and decisions by enabling them to identify, understand, and act to transform social relations and practices in which power is structured unequally." The social and political power of literacy can be seen clearly in an antialcohol literacy program developed in the state of Andhra Pradesh in India. A literacy program was established in a way that allowed the female participants to select their content focus. The women selected alcohol use, a serious issue facing their communities. As a result, the literacy program coalesced into a civic effort that successfully banned alcohol sales. The state, later realizing the loss of income from tax on alcohol, eliminated the literacy program and eventually allowed alcohol to be sold again.

Characteristics of People as Language Users

To frame the subsequent discussion of health and health literacy, the following key characteristics of people as language users are important to keep in mind:

• People are meaning makers, no matter their skill. Speakers and readers try to make meaning from what they read, see, and hear, as the following joke circulated on the internet in 2005 shows:

Q: Is your appearance here this morning pursuant to a deposition notice which was sent to your attorney?

A: No, this is how I dress when I go to work.

• Literacy and language reflect and influence how we see the world and make meaning. The way we use language and how literate we are says much about how we interpret the world. Consider the profound yet subtle distinction the speakers of English and the Hopi language make in the following utterance:

English: "I am riding the horse."

Hopi: "The horse is running for me."

The two utterances demonstrate uniquely different views of the relationship between people and animals.

Using a more contemporary example, after 9/11, militaristic and scientific language mingled and percolated into everyday language, reshaping our vocabulary and worldview. New words entered the public dialogue and consciousness. The noun *weapon* has been made into a verb, *weaponizing,* as in "weaponizing a substance," and "dirty bombs" do not refer to sanitation. Terrorist groupings became "cells"; *spores* became a word used to describe what might be in the mail. By November 2001, U.S. postal workers were being called "unlikely foot soldiers in the war against terror" (Cannon, 2001, p. 18).

• Literacy is a means to create social norms as well as a means to question these norms. Literacy permits local knowledge to be generalized. Therefore, literacy is in part about power, and its goal includes social transformation. For example, literacy programs have been linked with women's empowerment in microcredit programs. One such program is the Nepal Women's Empowerment Project (WEP) in which literacy improvement among women was combined with microfinance education. Over 100,000 women (native citizens) were taught how to read and write, how to start small businesses and village banks, and how to manage small health or social projects. With their knowledge and skill, they went on to teach other women. After three years, the number of women deemed literate rose from 39,000 to 122,000; the number of small businesses rose from 19,000 to 86,000, yielding income of more than $10 million; 1,000 village banks were founded; and 50,000 social projects were planned and carried out on self initiative (PACT Nepal, n.d.).

• People's literacy skills vary greatly. There is tremendous variability in people's literacy skills (reading, writing, numeracy, and speaking) and in their spoken language abilities. These skills can change over one's lifetime. Variation in literacy abilities is related to many factors, including education, socioeconomic status, culture, speech community, health status (such as sight and hearing impairments), cognitive and mental capacities, and relevance and motivation.

• Literacy is dynamic; it evolves. Over a lifetime, we can acquire literacy abilities to meet life's changing circumstances. Take, for example, the high school dropout who learns to read when 33 years old and is able to get a job not obtainable beforehand; the midlife mother who returns to the workforce and learns how to do a sales presentation using PowerPoint; or the 70-year-old woman who learns to communicate in chatrooms on the internet and finds an arthritis support group.

Wrapping Up

It is understandable that deficits become most salient when experts of any type need to communicate with nonexperts. In this chapter, we have introduced a discussion of the consequences of low health literacy in the United States. Low health literacy is an important public health issue that, if addressed, will greatly contribute to the health, safety, and well-being of millions of people.

In the next chapter, we briefly review the history of health education and promotion over the past century in the United States. The growing emphasis on health literacy has evolved from a long history of both successful and unsuccessful strategies of health promotion and health education. This historical lens will help the reader as subsequent chapters develop our model of health literacy.

Exercises

1. Choose a health situation appropriate to your practice or profession. List the types of decisions your patients or the public are asked to make in regard to this situation. Now list the types of skills that they need in order to make these decisions.

2. Choose a print communication (brochure, handout, fact sheet, ad, patient worksheet) that you use with patients or the public. Make two lists: one of elements that you believe your patient or other recipient would find easy

to read and use, the other containing elements that would be hard to read and use. Explain how you would address the complexity.

3. Discuss the opportunities and obstacles to enhancing shared decision making among patients and publics.

2

Advancing Health Literacy
Getting Here from There

An increasing body of evidence shows that health literacy is linked to health status: the more health literate an individual is, the healthier is the individual. This book demonstrates that health literacy principles and practices connect health promotion, education, and health delivery with improved patient and public health knowledge and decision making. To place that emerging understanding of health literacy in context, in this chapter we review the history of health education and promotion over the past century and set a foundation for readers to learn more about the role that health literacy plays in human health.

Historical Considerations

There is a long history of attempting to educate and promote better health. Urbanization, scientific discovery including advances in medical and communication technologies, and changes in the public health and public education systems all have significant impacts on individual perception and involvement in health and well-being.

It has always been important for health professionals to communicate effectively with laypeople. In the twentieth century, effective therapies and helpful disease prevention strategies emerged through scientific development. The growing understanding of disease and the precision of healing have accented the need for health professionals to communicate effectively with laypeople.

Populations sufficiently educated and empowered to understand and act on health messages also emerged in the twentieth century. The heterogeneity of the population in primary language, culture, educational attainment, access to information, and other considerations has amplified the communication challenge. The sciences of communication and human motivation developed, and health literacy, that is, the ability of people to understand and use medical and health information, emerged as an essential component of medical and public health practice.

Attempts to deliver health messages to people effectively, from sources both altruistic and avaricious, have proliferated in the past 200 years in the United States. Witch doctors were followed by patent medicine hucksters in the 19th century. Public health officials and nonprofit agencies assumed the task when federal legislation did away with the hucksters. The arrival of radio, television, and now the internet created new opportunities for communicators, particularly commercial advertisers. Marketing became a profession and a major force in society. The power of marketing techniques soon came to the attention of social researchers and activists who developed social marketing, employing marketing practices to address social issues such as health and the environment (McKenzie-Mohr & Smith, 1999).

In the twentieth century, chronic lifestyle diseases replaced infectious diseases as the dominant health threat. The civil rights and feminist movements empowered a larger segment of society; hierarchical, authoritarian constraints were weakened, and a previously submissive population of patients and clients began to demand a role in health care decision making. Informed consent was mandated by law. Managed care arrived, and insurance plans proliferated, making it ever more difficult to navigate the health care system.

A Brief History: How Did We Get to Health Literacy?

The growing emphasis on health literacy evolved from a long history of both successful and unsuccessful strategies of health promotion and health education. In many ways, changes in the understanding and methods of health promotion are about changing concepts of health by both consumers and providers. Urbanization, scientific discovery, advances in medical and communication technologies, and changes in the public education system, among other things, all significantly bear on individual perception and involvement in health and well-being. This brief history of health education and communication will prepare readers to see health literacy as the organizing framework bridging health promotion and education with greater patient and public health knowledge and informed decision making.

Our snapshot of health care during the past century begins with the patent medicine boom of the late 1800s and then moves to the tuberculosis epidemic of the early 1900s, continues to the polio epidemic of the mid-20th century, and concludes with a look at health needs and health promotion models in the late 20th century. Emerging from this short history are themes of how early regulation helped protect consumers and how a greater need for an informed public grew as medicine and society became more complex.

Patent Medicines

Patent medicines played an important role in health care throughout the 19th and into the early 20th century. Medical practice prior to the 20th century was primitive and unscientific, often more harmful than beneficial. It has been said that it was not until the early 20th century that the encounter of the average patient with the average doctor had a 50 percent chance of benefiting the patient. Unregulated until the beginning of the 20th century, patent medicine hucksters built a now forgotten empire of tonics and elixirs claiming health benefits. Most patent medicines, however, contained high amounts of alcohol or narcotics such as opium, which probably played the largest role in easing pain and anxiety. But because nostrum makers were not required to list ingredients, even people who swore by temperance were able to "benefit" from the remedies.

Lydia Pinkham's Vegetable Compound (Exhibit 2.1) was a well-known, well-marketed all-purpose tonic that women used during the

Exhibit 2.1. Nineteenth-Century Advertisement for Lydia Pinkham's Vegetable Compound.

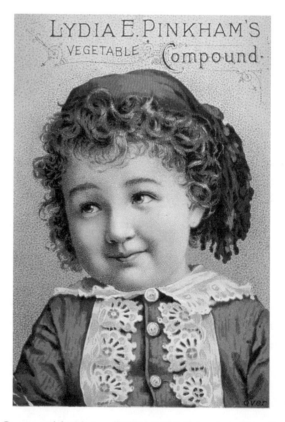

Source: Courtesy of the National Library of Medicine, http://wwwihm.nlm.nih.gov/ihm/images/A/21/049.jpg.

late 1800s (Young, 1985). This was a time when patent medicines were the drugs of choice, and patients were just as likely to look for relief from their ills from a local peddler as from a doctor. Many patients were dissatisfied with painful and unreliable treatments, such as bloodletting, employed by doctors of the day, and sought alternate therapies. In patent medicines they found a plethora of seemingly effective, less noxious treatments (Young, 1985).

Licensed doctoring had not come on the scene in the 19th century. There was no health insurance, and public health assistance was left to philanthropists. Pinkham advertised that "only a woman understands a woman's ills" (doctors were always men) and offered relief for all "female ailments." She encouraged her clients to write to her for advice and responded by urging them to use her compound and improve personal cleanliness. (Identifying a lucrative market in the half of the population excluded by her original marketing strategy, she eventually added "male complaints" to the compound's label. When kidney problems were identified as a popular threat, they too were added.)

The rise of patent medicines in England and the United States resulted from an increased desire for health care alternatives among consumers and shrewd marketing by enterprising individuals. Patent medicines took quick advantage of the development of the printing press in the mid-17th century and immediately began aggressive advertising campaigns. Word-of-mouth advertising was replaced by journal advertisements, and medicine sales increased exponentially (Young, 1985), setting the stage for a long history of direct-to-consumer pharmaceutical advertising that continues today, albeit legally in only a handful of countries.

Patent medicine makers were savvy marketers of their products. Attractive illustrations and colorful language increased sales, and trademarks improved product identification. Some labels were printed with pictures of famous people and places, while others boasted exotic concoctions of "Indian origin" (Young, 1988). Advertisements targeted cultural groups by running in multiple languages, a great appeal to the large immigrant population of the day (Carrigan, 1994). Producers targeted blacks with hair straightening creams and facial bleachers. The products were popular and publicized widely in the African American press. Patent medicine advertisements marked the beginning of health promotion efforts in emerging industrialized nations, a beginning of dubious origin.

Consumer Protection

The 1906 Food and Drug Act marked the beginning of the regulation of medication in the United States by setting nationally recognized standards on medicine safety, and later efficacy, and criminalizing false drug claims. The statute prevented the manufacture, sale, or transportation of misbranded, poisonous, or deleterious drugs and medicines. It enabled the government to go to court against illegal products but lacked affirmative requirements to guide compliance. It regulated drug concentrations, imitation drugs, and contents tampering and required that all narcotics in medicines be reported (Janssen, 1981). In addition, the act put severe restrictions on how patent medicines could be produced and sold, thus crippling the patent medicine industry. Simultaneously, scientific medicine was advancing.

By 1938, in the wake of the tragic death of 100 people (in 15 states across the country between September and October 1937) from a poisonous and unregulated elixir of sulfanilamide, the Federal Food, Drug, and Cosmetic Act was passed. This new act provided consumer protection by requiring scientific proof of the safety of new products, regulating therapeutic devices, making the prosecution of false drug claims easier, and raising the penalty for violators (Janssen, 1981).

In the late 1950s, the United States avoided certain tragedy to its populace by adhering to the 1938 drug legislation and putting on hold an application for the distribution of thalidomide, an anti–morning sickness pill. Between 1957 and 1962, the sale of thalidomide in Europe caused the deaths and deformity of more than 10,000 newborns of mothers who had used the drug during pregnancy. This tragedy prompted 1962 amendments requiring that adverse reactions of drugs be reported to the Food and Drug Administration, that risks and benefits of drugs accompany medical journal advertisements of drugs, and that the effectiveness, as well as the safety, of a drug be proven before it is marketed. These amendments removed thousands of prescription drugs from the market (Janssen, 1981).

Early Public Health Promotion and Education

At the start of the 20th century, the environmental conditions in which people lived changed dramatically with the rise in industrialization and urbanism. A consequence of these changes was increased exposure and transmittal of diseases. Public health increasingly focused on people's awareness of diseases and on teaching hygiene. Initially, philanthropic organizations, and later the federal government through state and local health departments, led this effort.

Tuberculosis: The Earliest Mass Public Education Effort in the United States

A reaction to the spread of tuberculosis in the early 20th century was the antituberculosis movement, or the "era of hygiene" (Paterson, 1950). The goal was to transform the health habits of individuals through increased public education about the disease and its spread (Starr, 1982). The approach to health promotion was predominantly command and control.

Traditional health education models assumed that the public lacked knowledge or was misinformed. They relied on information delivery or information transfer to address the health issue. Initially it was believed that physicians or public health overseers could simply transfer information to the public in much the same way that physicians inoculate a patient (Searle, 1969). For example, in 1895, the Pennsylvania Society began an antispitting campaign, and around the same time the Health Protective Association, a women's group, did its own tuberculosis prevention efforts by posting signs in factories that read, "Don't spit" (Price, 1952). Although their attempts to address the tuberculosis problem did not develop beyond this initial effort, they were evidence of a growing interest in health education (Shryock & Welch, 1957).

Two philanthropic organizations formed in the 1900s to combat two specific diseases were the National Tuberculosis Association (NTA) (later renamed the American Lung Association) and the National Foundation for Infantile Paralysis (NFIP) (later renamed March of Dimes). In their public health education work, these organizations arranged for wide distribution of educational materials that state agencies frequently could not afford to create. Furthermore, such agencies were both consultants and leaders, relied on by state agencies for their expertise (Gunn & Platt, 1945).

Among the NTA's most important public health education strategies was the start of multilevel campaigns employing radio, television (once available), newspaper, posters, leaflets, exhibits, and mobile diagnostic units to reach large groups of people. They were effective at that time for a specific disease whose remedy consisted of improvements in basic hygiene practices. By midcentury, however, diseases, medicine, and society were more complex and created the need for changes in strategies and models of health promotion and education.

Early Health Education Campaigns

The NTA TB campaign in 1904 was one of the earliest health education campaigns in the United States (Paterson, 1950). In 1907, the NTA launched the Christmas Seal Campaign to raise funds for an educational approach to combating tuberculosis. The stamps, which depicted a double-barred cross, were intended to symbolize the "stamp out" of tuberculosis (Exhibit 2.2). The sale of the annual seal helped to educate the public about tuberculosis by creating institutional value, being widely distributed, and increasing commitment among purchasers (Jacobs, 1940; Chadwick & Pope, 1946; Starr, 1982).

Exhibit 2.2. National Tuberculosis Society Christmas Seal Campaign, 1907.

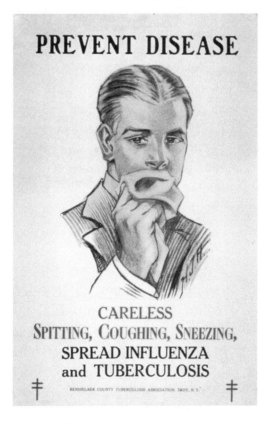

Education campaigns targeted labor, management, and ethnic groups where tuberculosis prevailed. The association also provided special training to physicians, nurses, technicians, and public health workers, and it encouraged health departments, sanatoria, and tuberculosis associations to use such trained professionals. It also made grants and fellowships available to help fund investigative studies regarding tuberculosis (National Tuberculosis Association, 1945; Perkins, 1952).

The campaigns proved successful in reaching the general public. For example, New York's Bureau of District Health Administration compared the results of mass X-ray tuberculosis campaigns by the health department in two city housing projects. The results showed that "where there was no previous education and promotional campaign by the voluntary agency only 5 percent of the residents took advantage of this important necessary service. Where the local district health committee provided a great deal of stimulation, education, and promotion of the mass X-ray, 40 percent cooperated with the Health Department and were X-rayed" (Gunn & Platt, 1945).

The NTA's work greatly contributed to the continuing decline in the tuberculosis death rate. In 1900, there were 194.4 deaths per 100,000 people. By 1920, the death rate had dropped to 113.1 per 100,000 (Paterson, 1950). The introduction of streptomycin in the mid-1940s and subsequent antituberculosis drugs also dramatically reduced the incidence and prevalence of tuberculosis in the United States.

Campaign Strategies

From the start of these early campaigns in the United States, a number of vehicles for getting the word out were used. There were newspapers in English and other languages and pamphlets for the public, teachers, nurses, and physicians (Shryock & Welch, 1957). The association issued nine pamphlets in its first 15 years, with titles including "How to Avoid Contracting Tuberculosis" and "How Persons Suffering from Tuberculosis Can Avoid Giving the Disease to Others." There were also exhibits displaying unhygienic surroundings, clean living situations, and sanatoriums (Shryock & Welch, 1957). The first of such displays was the 1905–1907 traveling exhibit that visited cities in the United States, Canada, and Mexico. More than 370,000 people viewed the exhibit. Another exhibit was launched in 1909 that was prepared in Spanish and taken to Puerto Rico. Nurses also played a vital role in public health education about tuberculosis, especially helpful with hard-to-reach populations. In order to reach people who did not attend clinics, it became necessary to take the mobile diagnostic facilities to the patient and family. Although expensive, this was deemed the most effective way to discover and control tuberculosis among specific groups in the community (Chadwick & Pope, 1946).

Targeting children, the "Modern Health Crusade" focused on childhood tuberculosis and stimulated public schools to create health service and health education programs (Jacobs, 1940). A child bought 10 cents worth of seals, became a member of the crusade, and received a small certificate. Children moved up an honor scale as they carried out hygiene-related chores, including brushing their teeth (Means, 1962; Shryock & Welch, 1957; Starr, 1982). By 1940, 25 million school children in the United States had received routine health instruction as part of their school curriculum (Jacobs, 1940).

What differentiates these early campaigns from health campaigns 50 years later is that less refined forms of targeting communication were understood and practiced. Campaigns worked with often unresearched, broad assumptions about the audience. There was virtually no attention to literacy level and subtle cultural variables.

National Foundation for Infantile Paralysis (March of Dimes)

As with the tuberculosis campaigns of the first quarter of the 20th century, health campaigns to combat infantile paralysis focused on education and behavior change. But now a more conscious focus on the recipient of the message, the public and patients, developed.

In 1915, there were fewer than 2,500 cases of infantile paralysis (poliomyelitis) reported in the United States. That number increased to almost 15,000 in 1945 and to more than 28,000 by 1951. The number of reported deaths from the disease rose from 661 in 1915 to 1,186 by 1945 (National Foundation for Infantile Paralysis, n.d., 1947).

The National Foundation for Infantile Paralysis (NFIP) was established in 1938 by President Franklin Delano Roosevelt, who had contracted the disease at the age of 39 (Cohn, 1955). From 1938 to 1958, the foundation focused on polio research, rehabilitation, and patient care. While NFIP funded scientists performing research in their laboratories, volunteers took on the responsibility of raising funds to support the research and implement education programs for polio victims and their families. Jonas Salk's vaccine for polio was licensed in 1955, and polio remained a threat until the population at large embraced vaccination.

As with tuberculosis, polio campaigns used a great number of local and national communication and education strategies. As medical research on polio advanced, public health promotion evolved from teaching about behaviors designed to prevent the disease (keeping children away from other unknown children), to explaining the vaccine clinical trials, and ultimately, and most important, to messages that encouraged inoculation of children. The "Polio Pledge" leaflet in the box is an example of a prevention message typical of the time.

Polio Pledge

If polio comes to my community:

- I will remember to:

    Let my children continue to play and be with their usual companions. They have already been exposed to whatever polio virus may be in that group, and they may have developed immunity (protection) against it.

- I will not:

    Allow my children to mingle with strangers, especially in crowds, or go into homes outside their own circle. There are three different viruses that cause polio. My children's group may be immune to one of these. Strangers may carry another polio virus to which they are not immune (National Foundation for Infantile Paralysis, 1952).

Promoting the Salk Vaccine Trials, 1953–1954

Over 1.8 million children participated in the polio vaccine trials. In many instances, children themselves took home the first piece of information about the trials to their parents and thus became the first "Polio Pioneers." These children received Polio Pioneer buttons and award cards (for those who were injected) at ceremonies covered by different media sources (National Foundation for Infantile Paralysis, 1954). The public education outreach regarding the trials was generally successful. According to a Gallup Poll reported on May 31, 1954, 90 percent of the population knew of the polio vaccine trials.

Getting the Right Message to the Right People,
at the Right Time, with the Desired Effect

The foundation's most significant campaign began in 1955 when the injectable Salk polio vaccine was deemed "safe, potent, and effective" for use. As a result, the NFIP launched a program of free vaccination for school children in the first and second grades. This age group was selected because of its high polio incidence and because it was easily accessible in schools (National Foundation for Infantile Paralysis, 1955). By the end of 1956, 45 million Americans had received one or more doses of the polio vaccine, and the incidence of polio had dropped 48 percent. In January 1958, the U.S. Public Health Service reported that 65 million people had received one or more Salk shots, and reported cases dropped more than 80 percent in two years (National Foundation for Infantile Paralysis, 1958a).

Targeting Audiences, Tailoring Messages

What truly distinguished these polio campaigns from earlier TB campaigns was the focus on the receivers, or target audiences. The newly emerging professions of advertising and marketing influenced health promotion efforts. Understanding the audience was on its way to becoming as important as the content of the message itself.

Radio Announcement Targeting Teenagers for Polio Shots

"Hey teens! How's your date calendar? If you live in [local] county, you better make your next date with your doctor" (National Foundation for Infantile Paralysis, 1958b).

Social Movements and Advocacy in the 1960s and 1970s

The civil rights movement, the women's movement, and the anti–Vietnam War movement, along with the growing consumer, self-help, and environmental justice movements, emerged during the 1960s and 1970s. These movements advocated for social justice and empowerment for both individuals and communities.

A "clear language" initiative began in the 1970s. Before the term *health literacy* was coined, public health professionals grew more concerned about helping consumers understand health information. The importance of consumer comprehension of health messages was formally highlighted in a Federal Trade Commission "plain English" project launched in 1970 (Bettman, 1975). The topic of the program was food safety, and the goal was to make messages easier for the public to understand and act on, but what happened was quite the opposite. Jacoby (1977), who studied the complexity of the messages developed, found that they were hard to understand and required "corrective advertising." This first glimpse into the mismatch between complex health information and the abilities of the general public did not come into sharper focus for another 10 years.

Informed Consumer Decision Making and Community Collaboration in the 1980s and 1990s

During these two decades, the complex relationships of health and sociocultural factors became even more of a reality. Top-down, command-and-control models of health promotion were proven ineffective in improving public health (Green, Lightfoot, Bandy, & Buchanan, 1985; Maibach & Parrott, 1995). More attention was given to analyzing and improving patient-physician interaction (Dickson, Hargie, & Morrow, 1989; Roter & Hall, 1992).

Early research into the linguistic and psychosocial aspects of patient-physician interaction yielded compelling findings about power relationships, complex language, and the intricacy of face-to-face encounters (Roter & Hall, 1989; Shapiro et al., 1983; Erzinger, 1991; Ong, de Haes, Hoos, & Lammes, 1995). Acknowledging (if not yet studying and understanding) the needs of patients and consumers became an important component of health promotion. Just as marketing research honed the ability to create markets through timely and targeted advertising, it was becoming clearer to health educators and communicators that consumer involvement was critical to whether a message was noticed and acted on (Evans & Clarke, 1983). As the formal study of the conscious and unconscious motivators of human decision making and behavior informed the commercial marketplace, this also trickled through to the study of health decision-making research and health promotion.

HIV/AIDS and other health problems, including the rise in substance abuse, low birth weight in infants, poor diets, and depression, to name a few, took tolls on personal health and the health and well-being of communities. These more chronic threats to health had, and continue to have, consequences for schools, workplaces, communities, and other social institutions, as well as economic consequences.

The HIV/AIDS epidemic highlighted the need for practical, relevant education. Outraged by public silence, grassroots organizations in major cities took on much of the early struggle to educate the public (Valdiserri, 2003). Greater emphasis was placed on community empowerment and shared decision making (Cancela, Chim, & Jenkins, 1998). The Institute of Medicine's (IOM) report *The Future of Public Health* (1988) called for a more inclusive societal lens through which to view the health and well-being of citizens.

With a growing understanding of these issues, in 1993 the Centers for Disease Control and Prevention (CDC) produced its first guidelines highlighting the importance of community planning. It noted that carefully targeted health messages seemed to be more effective than broad, general campaigns in terms of reaching meaningful health outcomes. The CDC (1998a) stressed that publicly funded HIV prevention programs "needed to improve in their ability to target interventions to those most at risk." As part of its "America Responds to AIDS" campaign, the CDC charged states with creating local public service announcements that would be appropriate for specific local audiences.

Some individuals and groups were increasingly attempting to acquire scientific and medical knowledge, as was demonstrated in at least three major health areas during the 1980s and 1990s: HIV/AIDS, breast cancer, and environmental toxicant contamination (Long Island Breast Cancer Coalition, n.d.; Brown & Mikkelsen, 1997; Epstein, 1995; Valdiserri, 2003). Activist, disease-based organizations have demonstrated that the lay public can learn and participate in scientific and medical dialogue and contribute to setting research and policy agendas. For example, the group 1 in 9: Long Island Breast Cancer Action Coalition demonstrates a model of lay expertise. In 1990, this group was founded by residents concerned about and outraged by the high incidence of breast cancer on Long Island and the lack of progress that had been made in addressing this issue. Its concerns about how environmental factors may be related to the cause and development of breast cancer helped change the role of women in the fight against breast cancer from inactive to proactive (www.1in9.org). Learning the science of the disease and contributing to the dialogue that propelled research and policy have made the Long Island Breast Cancer Action Coalition a model of community participation and the role of lay health experts.

Development of Models of Behavior Change

As traditional, top-down communication proved to be unequal to the task, targeted communications and social marketing grew in importance. Social marketing is a research-based process focusing on understanding the context and motivations of consumers. Its primary goal is to influence attitudes and behaviors by using marketing principles for social good rather than profit. Audience analysis, segmentation, and formative and evaluative research are the main components (Andreason, 1995; McKenzie-Mohr & Smith, 1999).

Social marketing approaches attempt to address these central questions to advancing public health (Louis & Sutton, 1991; McGuire, 1989):

- How do you get people's attention?

- What motivates people to change and adopt healthier behaviors?

- How do individual cognitive, psychological, and cultural factors influence health behaviors and health status?

A number of models of individual behavior and change theories developed at the same time. Social-cognitive approaches became popular as they focused on describing stages of change and pointed to ways to change individual health behaviors (Fischhoff, 1989; Prochaska & DiClemente, 1983; Prochaska, DiClemente, & Norcross, 1992). So too did the study of self-efficacy and its relationship to strengthening positive health attitudes and behaviors, and adopting healthier choices (Bandura & Cervone, 1983; Maibach & Parrott, 1995). Other behavior change theories include diffusion of innovations, health belief models, social influence, social comparison, social norm theories, and theories of reasoned action. This is an incomplete list of the many theories that attempt to explain human behavior and attitudes.

Managed Care and Health Insurance

During this same time, managed care models expanded, increasing the need for individuals to understand health insurance and the importance of knowledge and advocacy in accessing desired services and appealing benefit disputes. These skills are particularly challenging for many low-income families, immigrant and refugee families, the elderly, and less educated people. Many among the elderly, with some of the lowest literacy skills, are beneficiaries of Medicare but do not understand the basics of their coverage.

All the while, the number of uninsured rose, highlighting serious equity problems. According to the Urban Institute's National Survey of American Families, 41 million people were uninsured in the United States in 2001 (Blendon, Young, & Desroches, 1999). One out of every six adults and children under the age of 65 had no insurance. Younger low-income adults, particularly blacks and Hispanics, are most likely to be uninsured (Holahan & Brennan, 2000). A third of the uninsured have family incomes over twice the federal poverty level (Winterbottom, Liska, & Obermaier, 1995). States have become increasingly reliant on managed care programs to contain Medicaid costs and provide quality care. By 1998, more than half (54 percent) of the people on Medicaid were in managed care programs (Health Care Financing Administration, 1998). The rise of managed care and its own complexities required consumers to know more and be prepared to make choices about plans, providers, and costs.

The 21st Century

Over the past 100 years in the United States, there have been many changes in medicine and doctors, the roles and responsibilities of patients-turned-consumers, the privileging of science information and technology, and the role of community-level collaboration. In the 19th century and earlier, communicable diseases were predominant, and the population was generally less educated. As education levels rose, individuals became more capable of understanding the causes of disease. This led to an increased desire on the part of at least some individuals to participate in decision making. In the 19th century, health professionals made most decisions autocratically, and patients followed unquestioningly.

Contemporary society is quite different. Health instructions are no longer unchallenged, and dialogue is replacing monologue. Importantly, the predominant health problems have become chronic diseases largely related to lifestyle such as diet and exercise and require behavior changes for their prevention and treatment. Successful chronic disease management calls for collaboration among providers, public health officials, individuals, families, and communities.

Literacy and Health

There is a long history of investigating how individual capabilities and social processes explain or predict health. As demonstrated in major policy reports such as *Healthy People 2010* (U.S. Department of Health and Human Services, 2000), poor education, low literacy, poor health, and early death are strongly linked in the United States and around the rest of the world. These are particularly important areas of investigation, especially in the light of the trend evident since the beginning of the 20th century that most major advances in health are due to the application of new knowledge and technologies, such as immunizations and preventive medicine (World Bank, 2002).

Research demonstrates that low-literate individuals often cannot read medication labels accurately, may take medication incorrectly, may not understand consent forms, and generally have difficulty understanding print instructions for follow-up care and reading health advisories and warnings (World Education, 2004;

Nielsen-Bohlman et al., 2004; Schwartzberg et al., 2005). However, low ability to read and write (functional literacy) is not the only thing that contributes to low health literacy. Personal experience, cultural beliefs, access to medical information and health care systems, and much more can determine what people perceive, understand, and act on.

The 1992 National Adult Literacy Survey found that almost 50 percent of the adults in the United States read at the eighth-grade level or lower (Kirsch et al., 1993; Schillinger et al., 2002). Yet most health materials are written at levels far beyond the literacy abilities of a large segment of the population (Doak & Doak, 2002; Root & Stableford, 1999).

Health Literacy in the 21st Century

In the United States, individual health behavior currently has a far greater impact on rates of death and disability than biomedical advances (Institute for the Future, 2003, 2004). While the 20th century saw a dramatic decrease in death from communicable diseases, primarily thanks to antimicrobials and improved hygiene, the 21st century will likely see a dramatic increase in death and disability from chronic conditions, including heart disease and cancer, as well as mental health conditions and other illnesses related to lifestyle and behavior (Institute for the Future, 2003; see Figure 2.1). Roughly 100 million Americans live with a chronic illness or disability (LaForce & Wussow, 2001). Between 1990 and 2020, the absolute number of deaths from noncommunicable diseases is projected to increase by 77 percent (from 28.1 million to 49.7 million people). An estimated 50 percent of a person's health status will be attributable to lifestyle. Ineffective ways of paying for people's care and poor health care delivery systems make these statistics compelling. The following statistics are from the U.S. Department of Health and Human Services's publication "The Power of Prevention: Steps to a Healthier US Program and Policy Perspective" (2003):

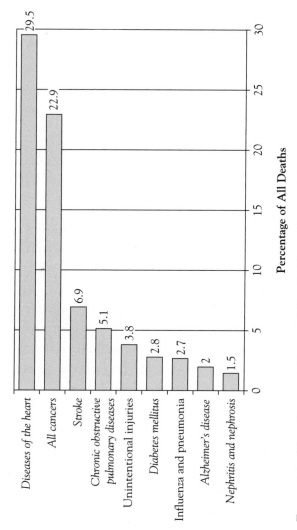

Figure 2.1. Most Common Causes of Death, United States, 2000.

Note: Italic type indicates chronic disease or condition.

Source: Department of Health and Human Services (2003). http://www.healthierus.gov/steps/summit/prevportfolio/power/index.html#we.

- More than 1.7 million Americans die of a chronic disease each year, accounting for about 70 percent of all U.S. deaths.

- Five chronic diseases—heart disease, cancer, stroke, chronic obstructive pulmonary disease (e.g., asthma, bronchitis, emphysema), and diabetes—cause more than two-thirds of all deaths each year.

- Chronic disease is not just an issue among older adults. One-third of the years of potential life lost before age 65 are due to chronic disease.

The developing picture of public health in the United States comes into stark clarity when we add to this the fact that 46 percent of American adults are functionally illiterate in dealing with the health care system (American Medical Association, 1999). Patient involvement in disease management and decision making will be central to addressing both chronic and acute health problems. This means that effective health promotion is needed to get the right message to the right people at the right time in order to educate and influence behavior and, ultimately, health status (Ratzan, 2001). Individualized tailored messages will play a greater role given advances in identifying key characteristics of patients and populations and using technology to customize messages (Kreuter, Farrell, Olevitch, & Brennan, 2000).

We are at a time in health promotion when there is an urgency to identify relevant characteristics of individuals and groups in order to design effective health messages and campaigns. The success of health promotion will turn on bridging the content of health promotion to the end users who have adequate health literacy skills.

Wrapping Up

In this chapter we placed the field of health literacy in historical and social context. Lessons from health promotion and education history demonstrate the importance of closing the gap between expert and lay knowledge. Our understanding of health literacy is dynamic and evolving, and this historical framework lays the foundation for concepts developed in the subsequent chapters.

In the next chapter, we elaborate on the definition of health literacy, placing it squarely at the center of four important domains of knowledge that people use to understand and act on health messages and information: fundamental literacy, science literacy, civic literacy, and cultural literacy.

Exercises

1. Patient participation in health care decisions has increased in recent years, supported by laypeople and health professionals. List the barriers to participation, and give specific examples.

2. It is required by law that patients give informed consent for medical or surgical treatment. "Informed" patients are increasingly arriving at their physician's office with their recommendations for treatment. Define *informed*. Are there degrees of being "informed," and if so, at what point is a patient sufficiently informed to make valid decisions?

3. How does social marketing differ from mere information transfer? Give examples of each.

3

Defining Health Literacy

In this chapter, we develop a multidimensional definition and model of health literacy that addresses the skills and abilities that a person uses to understand and act on health information. Then we demonstrate how health professionals can use the model to communicate more effectively and advance the public's health literacy.

Literacy: Defining Terms

Literacy and health literacy are not the same.

Most often when you hear reference to a person's literacy, this means a person's ability to read and write (this is referred to as fundamental or general literacy). The term *illiterate* refers to someone who has only the barest of language skills. The United Nations Educational Scientific and Cultural Organization (UNESCO) defines an illiterate person as someone "who cannot, with understanding, both read and write a short, simple statement on his everyday life" (2005, p. 418, based on their 1958 definition). The term *illiterate* is laden with social and political stigma and should be used cautiously, as it does not mean that a person cannot speak (sometimes fluently), think logically, or interpret other forms of nonprint information (Walter, 1999). It can be helpful to think of a functionally illiterate person as someone who cannot use print language to perform activities of daily living such as reading a bus schedule, reading a prescription label, or doing basic math calculations to keep a checkbook (Kirsch, Junegeblut, Jenkins, & Kolstad, 1993).

Health literacy refers to people's abilities to understand and use health information, most often in print. The term *health literacy* as it is currently used in the United States does not distinguish clearly between health information in print and in spoken language or in other forms of written symbols: numbers, pictures, graphics, or other visual representations. In fact, modes of language (print, spoken, numbers, visuals) are often used rather interchangeably when people talk about health literacy.

Reality Bytes

The ways in which people notice, understand, and use health information are complex and defy simple formulas. They are central to our framework.

Reality 1: Fundamental Literacy and Health Literacy Are Different Capacities

A person can have high fundamental literacy but have low or insufficient health literacy and vice versa. Here are just a few examples:

- A college graduate with a degree in physics does not understand that taking multiple over-the-counter medications at once can be harmful.

- A retired librarian does not understand how Medicare works.

- A single mother with less than a sixth-grade education understands how to manage her four-year-old son's chemotherapy regimens and asks specific questions about his most recent blood counts.

Reality 2: How People Understand Health Messages Varies

There is tremendous variability in how people understand health messages. This competence is always changing and is influenced by many factors. To demonstrate this variability in people's understandings, we look at how three people respond to the antibiotic resistance print ad shown in Exhibit 3.1.

The ad meets many of the criteria for a high-quality communication: the visual is compelling and the lead message is hard hitting. But how well do consumers understand the content? The interviews we conducted (December 2003) elicited the following responses to it:

• An active, educated, high-literate, 73-year-old woman explains what the ad means to her as she browses the magazine: "I don't know. Is it saying that you don't have an infection when you're feeling so terrible? I don't understand the difference between

Exhibit 3.1. Antibiotic Resistance Print Ad.

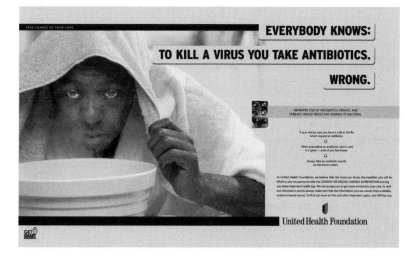

Source: United Health Foundation (2003).

having a virus and having a bacteria in me. I don't know if that makes sense. Maybe infections are only caused by bacteria. Could be." Either way, she reports that if she were feeling as "awful as that fellow [in the ad] I'd ask my doctor to put me on an antibiotic." When asked what "evidence based" means, she responds, unsure, "Probably they have to test you for cultures."

- A savvy, college-educated, high-literate, 39-year-old suburban mother reads the ad and says that "evidence based" means "whatever doctors do to test for that [bacteria]."

- A young postgraduate gets annoyed that the ad does not make clear that there is a difference between a virus and a bacterium: "And, you shouldn't have to tell people to 'never request' [that] your doctor shouldn't give you what you don't need." She defines "evidence based" as the "scientific trials as opposed to homeopathic stuff."

One can certainly argue that you do not need to understand "evidence based" to understand the central message: do not take antibiotics if you do not need them. But in the advertisement, that important central message is presented in complex language: "Improper use of antibiotics creates and spreads highly resistant strains of bacteria." The difficult words are *improper, resistant strains*, and perhaps *bacteria*. Some readers will miss the important relationship between individual behavior and the collective good, potentially furthering the creation of resistant strains of bacteria.

Reality 3: Health Literacy Is Productive and Generative

Health literacy is much more than understanding a finite list of health facts or vocabulary. Health literacy consists of a dynamic group of productive and generative skills a person calls on when facing new situations. This generativity is what makes health literacy sustainable and enables health-literate people to make more informed decisions, benefit from healthier choices, and have degrees of independence from experts and knowledge intermediaries. When people have a good degree of health literacy, they know how to seek out, access, judge, and use information about their health. They also are better prepared to know what they can discard as outdated, unreliable, or simply wrong.

Take, for example, using the internet to seek out health information. When we unpack the many layers of skills needed to use the web effectively, we see a long list, including these skills:

- Realizing the relevant information may be available on the internet

- Operating a computer and navigating the web

- Reading and comprehending the language used

- Determining the reliability of the information provider

- Being able to refer to or recall this information when seeking the advice of physicians or other experts

- Judging among and balancing those various sources of information to make an informed decision

A key aspect missing from many models of health literacy has been the importance of this generative nature of health literacy. This allows individuals to apply existing knowledge and skills to novel situations as they develop. In other words, a health-literate person knows how to handle the next problem, one never seen before. (This idea is discussed further later in this chapter.)

The Evolving Field of Health Literacy

The young and multidisciplinary field of health literacy emerged from two expert groups: physicians and other health providers and health educators, and adult basic education (ABE) and English for speakers of other languages (ESOL) practitioners. Physicians are a source of groundbreaking patient comprehension and compliance studies (Davis, Crouch, Wills, Miller, & Abdehou, 1990; Gazmararian, 1999; Parker, Baker, Williams, & Nurss, 1995; Roter, 1984; Schillinger et al., 2002; Williams et al., 1995; Williams, Baker, Parker, & Nurss, 1998). Adult basic education/English for speakers of other languages (ABE/ESOL) specialists study and design interventions to help people develop reading, writing, and conversation skills and increasingly infuse curricula with health information to promote better health literacy. A range of approaches to adult education brings health literacy skills to people in traditional classroom settings, as well as where they work and live (Doak et al., 1996; Hohn, 1997; National Center for the Study of Adult Learning and Literacy, n.d.; Muro, n.d.; Root & Stableford, 1999; Rudd, Zacharia, & Daube, 1998; World Education, 2004; Zarcadoolas et al., 2004). (See the links at WorldEd, http://www.worlded.org/us/health/lincs, and "A Selection of Health Literacy Articles and Research," published by Partnership for Clear Health Communication: http://www.askme3.org/pdfs/bibliography.pdf.)

Making Medical Language Clear and Simple

The field of health literacy has adopted a dominant strategy to tackle low health literacy: simplifying health and medical information. As early as 1974, the Federal Trade Commission, looking at nutritional information disclosures, provided evidence concerning the limitations of consumers' understanding of health information. Experts proposed that "plain English" be used in remedial messages about nutritional information (Bettman, 1975; Evans & Clarke, 1983; Jacoby, 1977). In general, the "plain language" or "clear and simple" movement within the field of health literacy focuses on adjusting health messages to match the low fundamental literacy level of patients and consumers (American Medical Association Foundation, 2003; Doak et al., 1996; Environmental Protection Agency, 1999; U.S. Food and Drug Administration, 2003; McGee, 1999; National Cancer Institute, 1994; Partnership for Clear Health

Communication, 2003; Root & Stableford, 1998). (The antecedents of the current simplicity movement date back to the 1960s when reading researchers assumed that if the content of a text fell outside a reader's specialty, the reader would prefer a simplified style of writing; Klare, 1963.) A basic goal of the clear language or simplification model is to get clear messages to the intended audience. The first passage that follows is difficult to read. The second one shows a simplification approach:

> *Hard to read [emergency room use]:* Going to the emergency room is a covered expense if you are experiencing conditions that are so serious that any reasonable person could assume that these conditions are life threatening. Acceptable conditions include: trouble breathing, heavy bleeding, or chest pain.

> *Easier to read:* Not all emergency room visits will be covered by your health plan. If you go to the emergency room because you have a serious, life-threatening condition, then this visit will be covered. Serious life-threatening conditions mean things like trouble breathing, heavy bleeding, or chest pain. If you go to the emergency room and the condition is not very serious, you will have to pay for the visit.

The second passage is easier to read because it uses simple vocabulary and simple sentences instead of complex structures, repeats key phrases, and defines terms.

Health Literacy: Making Health Sustainable

A reliable body of research demonstrates that patients with low fundamental literacy skills (reading, writing, and math) follow medical regimens less well than more literate patients. Because there is such a gap between the complexity of health information coming from the medical, scientific, and policymaking communities and the comprehension abilities of diverse publics, researchers and practitioners have focused on the surface level of people's understanding, that is, the vocabulary and the sentences. This focus leads to some important questions about patient understanding. For example, does the patient know how to read the directions for taking medications, and if not, how can those directions be simplified? Do at-risk groups understand radio messages about the importance of having a flu shot, and if not, how can those messages be clearer? Can diabetes patients do the math calculations required in home diet logs, and if not, how can more social math (user-friendly examples in place of complex numbers) be substituted for greater patient comprehension?

Although these questions are important and necessary, they are not sufficient to fully describe, build on, or improve a person's health literacy. The gap between the fundamental literacy of patients and other citizens and the reading level of health information alone is not sufficient to explain the complex skills involved in being health literate. The focus on simplifying surface-level language has backgrounded important sociocultural aspects of people's understanding and minimized the intricate, efficient, and inefficient strategies people have for comprehending and making health decisions.

The biomedical and psychological approach to health literacy dominant in the 1980s and 1990s often depicted individuals as lacking, or "suffering" from, low health literacy; assumed that recipients are passive in their possession and reception of health literacy; and believed that models of literacy and health literacy are politically neutral and universally applicable (Street, 1993a, 1993b). This approach is found lacking when placed in the context of broader ecological approaches to health. Ecological models propose connections between health literacy and a range of social, cultural, and environmental (built and natural) determinants of health and generally view health literacy as an issue for health providers, health educators and communicators, adult education, and the public alike (Zarcadoolas, Pleasant & Greer, 2005; Nutbeam, 1999; Kickbusch, 2001; Kerka, 2003).

This more robust view of health literacy includes the ability to understand scientific concepts, content, and health research; skills in spoken, written, and online communication; critical interpretation of mass media messages; navigating complex systems of health care and governance; and knowledge and use of community capital and resources, as well as using cultural and indigenous knowledge in health decision making (Curran, 2002; Nutbeam, 2000; Ratzan, 2001; Zarcadoolas et al., 2002).

A recent and emerging understanding is that health literacy serves both personal and societal functions. Health literacy is as much a public health issue as it is the challenge of individual patients (Kickbusch, 1997; Muro, n.d.; Nutbeam & Kickbusch, 2000; Ratzan, 2001; Rudd, 2002). A health-literate person is able to make better health decisions and benefit from healthier lifestyle choices; in addition, a health-literate individual can better participate in the "social, economic and environmental determinants of health, and be directed towards the promotion of individual and collective actions which may lead to modification of these determinants" (Nutbeam, 1999, p. 49).

As with any field on the move, there are periods of transitional development where research informs movement from old to new. We believe that understanding health literacy is not very well articulated among many health literacy experts. Questions such as the following are important:

- What factors besides reading make up health literacy skills?

- What sociocultural characteristics help define health literacy?

- Are there core health concepts that go into making a health-literate person?

- What are the limitations of simplifying health messages and materials? For example, when is plain language not so plain?

- What role do the media play in creating health literacy?

- How can understanding the mechanisms of health literacy assist health professionals to advance the public's health?

Many Types of Literacy Combine to Form Health Literacy

The questions above (and many more) lead to a new model for understanding health literacy that engages a broad range of skills and competencies. For example, as indicated in the following example, merely simplifying the reading level of a message does not necessarily make it more understandable to the consumer.

Consider the first sentence in a notice from a health insurer: "Due to the fact that this drug is not on our formulary we are denying your claim for reimbursement." We can apply the principles of plain language and rewrite the sentence—"We deny [or "will not pay"] your claim" or "We are denying your claim because this drug is not on our list of approved medications"—but the complexity of the concepts remains. To understand the main propositions in the "simplified" version of the message, the reader has to know something about the following concepts:

- The insurance company has the authority to pay or not pay bills. It does not automatically pay for any service or medication even if the doctor recommends it.

- Insurers use a finite (and often changing) list of allowable medications that they will and will not pay for.

- Not all medicines are the same.

To a greater or lesser degree, consumers must understand that in the circumstances of a denied claim, they can:

- Request an appeal

- Speak to their doctor about an alternative medication and treatment options

- Think about changing health plans

- Become an advocate for health care reform

To understand the message and know what to do to receive an affordable medication (one that is covered by health insurance), consumers need several types of literacy in several domains: they need to understand something about science and medicine, civic structures, and cultural norms.

A New Definition of Health Literacy

We define *health literacy* as the wide range of skills and competencies that people develop over their lifetimes to seek out, comprehend, evaluate, and use health information and concepts to make informed choices, reduce health risks, and increase quality of life.

Health literacy, like any other competency, is on a continuum. There is no on and off switch. A health-literate person is able to use health concepts and information generatively, applying information to novel situations. A health-literate person is able to participate in the ongoing public and private dialogues about health, medicine, scientific knowledge, and cultural beliefs. Health literacy evolves over one's lifetime and, like most other complex human competencies, is affected by health status as well as demographic, sociopolitical, psychosocial, and cultural factors. Thus, the benefits of health literacy impact the full range of life's activities: home, work, society, and culture (Rudd & Kirsch, 2003; World Health Organization, 1986).

A Multidimensional Model of Health Literacy

Our definition of health literacy is the foundation for a multidimensional model built around four central domains: fundamental literacy, scientific literacy, civic literacy, and cultural literacy. Literacy skill in one domain can contribute to developing literacy skill in another domain, and competencies in one area can compensate for a lack of competencies in another.

Fundamental literacy (reading, writing, speaking, and numeracy) refers to the ability to read, write, speak, and work with numbers. It is a keystone of health literacy for a number of reasons:

- Reading, writing, speaking, and computing are fundamental ways people develop skills, acquire information, and conduct daily life.

- Written and spoken health information is full of complex language (vocabulary and syntax).

- Health information and materials are often not tailored to end user skills and abilities in reading, writing, speaking, and numeracy.

Scientific literacy refers to the skills and abilities to understand and use science and technology, including some awareness of the process of science. We specifically include:

- Knowledge of fundamental scientific concepts

- Ability to comprehend technical complexity

- An understanding of technology

- An understanding of scientific uncertainty and that rapid change in the accepted science is possible

Civic literacy refers to skills and abilities that enable citizens to become aware of public issues, participate in critical dialogue about them, and become involved in decision-making processes. We include:

- Media literacy skills

- Knowledge of civic and governmental systems and processes

- Knowledge of power, inequity, and other hierarchical relationships

- Knowledge that personal behaviors and choices affect others in a larger community and society

Cultural literacy refers to abilities to recognize, understand, and use the collective beliefs, customs, worldview, and social identity of diverse individuals to interpret and act on information (Kreps & Kunimoto, 1994). Cultural literacy should be bilateral, in that the communicator (doctor, scientist, public health official) should understand aspects of the culture of the recipient (interlocutor), and the recipient should understand aspects of the professional culture of the sender.

Now we will take a closer look at these domains.

Fundamental Literacy: Reading, Writing, Speaking, and Numeracy

Using some complex information is inevitable in educating about a disease, medications, diagnostic procedures, or treatment options, as well as the intricacies of the health care system itself. For example, starting in 2003, states were required to disseminate information about protected health information. Although the following "Notice of Privacy Practices," required in the United States by the Health Insurance Portability and Accountability Act of 1996 (HIPAA), is written at approximately the 12th- to 15th-grade reading level, the language and concepts are ambiguous to even the best of readers:

> Protected health information (PHI) is individually identifiable health information, including demographic information collected from you or created or received by a heath care provider, a health plan, your employer, or a health care clearinghouse, and that relates to: (i) your

past, present, or future physical or mental health or condition; (ii) the provision of health care to you; or (iii)
the past, present or future payment for the provision of
health care to you [Blue Cross/Blue Shield of Rhode
Island, n.d., p. 1].

For many people, medical information and health system information are high barrier—hard to read and use. For low-literate
adults (reading at the fifth- to eighth-grade level), this material is
extremely difficult and will not advance their understanding of the
health issues, health systems, or their rights and responsibilities.

Example: Comparing and Choosing a Health Plan

Louise, who reads at about the fifth-grade level, receives a health
plan comparison chart and is trying to use it to help choose the right
plan for her family. The chart is meant to compare the benefits offered
by three health plans. There are eight benefit areas on the chart.
When Louise is asked how many health plans the chart is comparing, she responds, "Twenty-four health plans." She literally counted
the number of boxes across and down to reach this answer.

Louise's reading skills are not developed to the point that she
knows she should first read down the left-hand column where it tells
which health plans she is comparing. Then she should read from left
to right across each row to see what services and benefits each plan
covers. Finally, she should compare and contrast these benefits
to see which plan is best for her. This example demonstrates that fundamental literacy involves negotiating the meaning of words and sentences as well as navigating the many formats that messages can take.

Scientific Literacy

Ever more complicated medical technologies and continuing advances in science require individuals to have some science understanding. However, research into the public understanding of and
engagement with science reveals low levels of knowledge about sci-

ence (Dierkes & von Grote, 2000; Laugksch, 2000; Pardo & Calvo, 2002; Pleasant et al., 2003). The need for scientific literacy is illustrated in the following examples and further explicated in case studies presented in Chapters 7 to 12.

Example: Responding to Changing Medical Recommendations

Margaret, a 57-year old college-educated banker, has been on hormone replacement therapy (HRT) for seven years and believes it is safe and beneficial to her health. One day she hears the following on the radio: "Researchers today released a report that links HRT, which millions of women around the globe take, to ovarian cancer." Furthermore, the report states, "Recent trials that randomly assigned women to HRT or a placebo" have found that women on HRT are at an increased risk for heart attack or stroke.

Margaret's scientific literacy comes into play and interacts with the other domains of health literacy. Here are three possible levels of her literacy in this area:

Poorest health literacy: Margaret is never told, or does not understand, that the pills she takes are HRT.

Poor health literacy: Margaret hears this news with some exasperation and concludes that scientists are always finding out that they do not know what they thought they knew, so she ignores the finding and continues her HRT without discussing this latest report with her physician.

Better health literacy: Margaret understands that scientists and medical people make decisions and dispense guidelines and advice based on the best available scientific understanding at the time and that scientific evidence, like life experience, can be contradictory but is best interpreted in the aggregate rather than through individual studies or experiences. She decides to call her doctor to discuss her protocol specifically and sets out to learn more about the HRT controversy herself.

Like many other decisions in life, health decisions must be made on the best information available at the moment rather than ignore the information to await a never-arriving utopian world where all medical information is known and immutable.

In the following example, the words and sentences about diabetes are fairly easy to read, but the concepts behind the words require a more advanced level of scientific literacy. This again demonstrates that health literacy is the product of more than just understanding the vocabulary used in health care and medicine.

Example: Diabetes

According to the American Diabetes Association (n.d.), "Diabetes is a disease in which the body does not produce or properly use insulin. Insulin is a hormone that is needed to convert sugar, starches, and other food into energy needed for daily life. The cause of diabetes is a mystery, although both genetics and environmental factors such as obesity and lack of exercise appear to play roles" (para. 1).

This description contains difficult words (*insulin, hormone, properly, convert,* and *environmental*), and the last sentence is difficult to read because it combines three ideas within a long and complex clause structure; the main sentence is interrupted by additional ideas. But there is more complexity in this passage than at the word and sentence level.

If you unpack the content, looking for assumed concepts (what a reader or listener may have to understand), you can better appreciate how health literacy includes scientific literacy. Here are some of the scientific concepts embedded in the passage:

- The human body, much like a factory, produces chemical compounds, and these compounds regulate body functions.

- Food is converted to energy within the body and used.

- Some biological processes are poorly understood.

- Human health can be influenced by factors such as genetics, environment, and behaviors.

In discussing health literacy and where it intersects with scientific literacy, important questions are:

- What science must a person know to comprehend and decide to act on a specific health message?

- What assumptions about the listeners' scientific literacy are made by developers of health messages?

Civic Literacy

Health issues today are complex and require community-level responses as well as responses from institutional health providers and individuals. This is especially true with population-wide conditions such as childhood obesity, population-wide hazards such as environmental pollution, and population-wide threats such as bioterrorism and possible flu pandemic. Civic literacy refers to abilities that enable citizens to become aware of health issues through civic and social channels and become involved in the decision-making process.

The World Health Organization (WHO) defines community health broadly as "encompassing all of the environmental, social, and economic resources as well as the emotional and physical capacities, that enable people in a geographic area to realize their aspirations and satisfy their needs" (Lasker & Weiss, 2003, p. 18). Social capital and social cohesion models contribute to our understanding of the importance of people accessing and being able to make use of all types of networks within their community, from kinship networks and neighborhood associations to institutional networks (Cottrell, 1977; O'Connor, Parker, & Oldenburg, 2000). The personal and collective perception and experience of inequity plays a role in civic literacy as well; however, the mechanisms of influence are unresearched and poorly understood in the field of health literacy (LaVeist, 2002).

Social capital is another important aspect of civic literacy. Social capital is defined as "the resources embedded in social relations among persons and organizations that facilitate cooperation and collaboration in communities" (Gittell & Vidal, 1997, p. 16; Putnam, 2000). Social capital is at work through communities, networks, and institutions and has been studied for many years as an important aspect of understanding and improving human welfare, poverty amelioration, and economic development, especially in less industrialized countries (Coleman, 1990; Collier, 1998; World Bank, 1999; Putnam, 1995). The role of connections between people and communities has received scant attention in epidemiology and public health. For example, Koopman and Lynch (1999) showed that differing connections among people can produce significantly different patterns of infectious disease in a population. Only since the late 1990s, however, has social capital theory gained recognition in our understanding of public health (Wilkinson, 1996; Kawachi, Kennedy & Prothrow-Stith, 1997; Muntaner, Lynch & Smith, 2003). There is much need to learn more about the interplay of social capital and health literacy.

Given the ubiquitous and decentralized nature of health information in so many different media, a significant aspect of civic literacy involves critical understanding of the media and how health information is packaged and disseminated in TV, radio, print, and the internet.

Civic literacy allows an individual to better judge whom in society to trust and to better decide to act with the collective good in mind (Gaventa, 1993; Kawachi & Berkman, 1998). When people have a sense of both individual and collective identity, they are better prepared to consider and coordinate personal and collective interests. Civic literacy comprises a range of understandings, including:

- Judging the sources of information

- Judging the quality of information

- Knowing where and how to access information

- Knowing how to advocate for oneself and others

- Understanding the relationship between one's actions and the larger social group

The following example is a simple demonstration of understanding that personal actions can have broader health consequences.

Example: Civic Literacy Skills

The parent in this example is asked to act for the greater good of the school population through this note sent home from his child's day care: "It is now flu season. We want all our children at Willow Lane to stay healthy and be healthy in the coming months. Please be sure that you let us know if your child is home with the flu. We ask you to please not send your child to school if he or she has a cold or seems to be sick that morning. We look forward to your cooperation as well as a healthy and happy winter season."

One central proposition is that civic literacy allows the parent to understand and agree that the greater good of the class (and the school) is served if a sick child is kept home, regardless of the personal inconvenience.

A critical area requiring civic literacy is interpreting information in the media and on the internet.

Media and the Internet

Messages, reliable and unreliable, abound in our cultural media: TV, radio, newspapers, magazines, and the internet. For example, prescription drug advertising directed to consumers (rather than physicians) is an enormous business, with over $2.5 billion spent in 2000 (Frank, Berndt, Donahue, Epstein, & Rosenthal, 2002). This money has an impact. In a 2002 Food and Drug Administration (FDA) survey, 92 percent of physicians said patients had initiated a discussion of direct-to-consumer marketed drugs (Aikin, 2002). Furthermore, direct-to-consumer pharmaceutical advertising has increased the sale of specific medications. Physicians prescribe on the recommendation of patients (Hollon, 2005).

Civic literacy plays a critical role in consumers' ability to attend to and interpret the barrage of direct-to-consumer advertising of medications and treatment options. Health-literate consumers are aware of the source of the information and the potential biases of that source. Some of these are somewhat obvious, such as the advertisement of medications by their manufacturers. In direct-to-consumer pharmaceutical advertising, for instance, self-interested or biased "authorities" can present medical information in such a manner as to bias, or at the least persuade, the consumer or patient (see Chapter 4). The purpose is to sell a product rather than provide objective information. That is not to say that the information they present is necessarily false; rather, it is selective, emphasizing the positive aspects of the medication and deemphasizing the negatives. Little research is available on the literacy and health literacy demands of such advertising or the impact on low-literate consumers (Kaphingst et al., 2004a, 2004b).

Cultural Literacy

Culture refers to the shared and dynamic characteristics of a group of people, which may include language, patterns of behavior, beliefs, customs, traditions, and other modes of expression. These characteristics enable group members to have and communicate shared meanings. People use collective beliefs, customs, worldview, and social identity in order to interpret and act on health information. Culture is not static, but rather is ever changing and affected by factors including personal experience as well as larger group acculturation.

Cultural literacy enables individuals and institutions to respond respectfully and effectively to people of all cultures, classes, races, ethnic backgrounds, and religions in a manner that understands, affirms, and values their differences and protects and preserves the dignity of each (Sen, 1999; DiversityRX, 2005). Cultural literacy also refers to an understanding of the power of cultural practices to influence the health status of individuals as well as how they define a healthy lifestyle.

Awareness and skills in cultural literacy on the communicator's part can help frame health information to accommodate powerful cultural understandings of health information, science, and individual and collective action (Kreps & Kunimoto, 1994).

The word *culture* is often associated with "foreign born"—referring to people with religious and ethnic beliefs not shared by the larger, mainstream population. Unfortunately, the word often conjures up stereotypes that mask the complexity of culture and individuals. In terms of its role in health literacy, we must consider culture through a much broader lens. Thus, *culture* refers to how people identify themselves and with whom they identify in terms of values, perceptions, and actions. Examples include the culture of teenagers and their collective confidence in their immortality, the culture of the elderly who grew up in a "doctor-knows-best" milieu, the culture of the rural poor versus the urban poor, the culture of the internet and health chatrooms. This way of seeing culture is best understood by marketers and social marketers who tailor their messages to critical aspects of sense of self and collective identity. Health messages are comprehensible and effective when they are consistent with and speak to cultural beliefs and culturally driven behaviors.

In health communication, when we think of culture, we must consider the role of native country, native language, and ethnic beliefs. Over 46 million people (more than 17 percent of the current population in the United States) speak a language other than English at home. The way culture impacts individual health is poignantly captured in Anne Fadiman's account (1997) of a Cambodian family living in California and dealing with the health system as they try to treat their gravely ill child (*The Spirit Catches You and You Fall Down*). The family's culture frames how they understand medicine and treatment. Things many Westerners would take as easily understood, for example, directions to "take a tablespoon," often yielded questions like, "What is a tablespoon?" Hmong patients would not swallow a medication because it was "an inauspicious color."

"Whatever the prescription, the instructions on pill bottles were interpreted [by Hmong patients] not as orders but as malleable suggestions. Afraid the medicines designed for large Americans were too strong for them, some Hmong cut the dosage in half; others double-dosed so they would get well faster" (p. 70).

A patient whose culture does not have a model for chronic diseases may perceive similar episodes of illness in the past as unrelated: that is, a distinct illness, having distinct causes and cures. Similarly, some cultures feel that informing a patient of potential medical risk can influence outcomes or be dangerous to the patient (DiversityRX, 2005).

Ideally, cultural literacy is practiced at the individual, practitioner, and organizational levels (U.S. Department of Health and Human Services, Health Resources and Services Administration, 2004). In communication between provider and patients, for example, the sender (provider) understands important aspects of the culture of the receiver, and the receiver understands important aspects of the professional and scientific culture of the sender.

Integrating the Literacies

Integrating cultural literacy into a definition of health literacy that acknowledges the important roles of fundamental, science, and civic literacy produces a model that creates a road map for improving health communication and education activities:

- Analyzing the complexity of existing health information and materials

- Writing and designing more accessible information and materials

- Developing assessment tools that will create useful profiles of people's health literacy

- Conducting needs assessment for practitioners and organizations for improving communications and thus advancing public health literacy

Wrapping Up

In this chapter we have presented a model for understanding health literacy. We have shown that literacy and health literacy are much more than being able to read and write, although in achieving health literacy, spoken and written language are major currencies. The following chapter presents fundamentals of language and how it works in written and spoken messages.

Exercises

1. Review a health message or campaign, either spoken, print, media, or web based. List the assumptions it makes about the patient's or consumer's health literacy. Indicate which domains of health literacy these assumptions reflect.

2. Is there a list of minimum health literacy concepts you think apply to most patients? What would be on that list? Discuss the efficacy of creating such a list.

3. Pick a target population, and develop a health message designed with the four key domains of health literacy in mind.

4

Literacy at Work

In Chapter 3, we demonstrated an expanded model of health literacy. We also showed how complex much health communication can be. The good news is language is a flexible system, providing us with lots of ways to make meaning. An implication for health professionals is that we have great flexibility in the resources we can use to create effective health messages, promotions, and campaigns. This chapter presents some fundamentals of language and how it works in written and spoken messages.

How Language Works

Having a message doesn't guarantee you're communicating. In health promotion, we often think the content equals the message: "Smoking is a health hazard." "To control your blood sugar, you should eat a well-balanced diet." "The threat of a biological attack is remote." In this simplistic model of communication, the speaker delivers a message, "quit smoking," to a listener, who then acquires the intended meaning of the message. The schematic below demonstrates this one-way, unidimensional model of communication:

Speaker → Message → Listener

But effective health communication involves more than delivering a message from a sender (a physician or other expert) to a receiver (a patient or the public). The sender and receiver must intend to communicate and have some agreement on the ground rules. Each must know something about each other's context, circumstances, needs for information, and abilities to comprehend that information. Each must choose methods and channels of communication both can access and use easily. Table 4.1 is an elaboration of a widely accepted functional model of communication (Jakobsen, 1978): the scaffolding of communication architecture.

A successful message is one that is shared between the sender and the receiver, the success of that being contingent on this scaffolding having sufficient bricks and mortar.

As the model proposes, in addition to a message, you need a means of contact: oral, visual, print, TV, internet, art, or something else. You need to know something about the code: the rule-governed language of print, spoken, visual communication. The context is the setting: a doctor's office, a TV interview, a public meeting with health officials, or a web site, for example. The context can also be the life circumstances and psychosocial and cultural characteristics of the participants. For instance, telling a frightened public about anthrax is a much different context from announcing to a healthy pregnant woman that she is about to have twins. There are also shared rules—that is, codes of use—about what you can and cannot do in communication. For example, depending on the context, the patient is

Table 4.1. The Scaffolding of Communication Architecture.

Addresser	Message	Addressee
Speaker	Contact	Listener
Context	Code	Code
Code	Context	Context

permitted (and often encouraged) to ask questions, but it would be far less appropriate for a patient to instruct the doctor about a medical fact. An advertiser selling sneakers can bluntly instruct the consumer to "Just Do It," but this message might be outside the code of what a public health official might say to urge an elderly population to get a flu vaccination.

The components of communication can shift in emphasis as well. For example, you can focus on the receiver by using a check to see if the receiver understands: "Okay? Any questions so far?" Or you can focus on the message itself, such as in the cigarette packaging and the more graphic TV ads about the health risks of cancers now being used in countries such as Canada, the United Kingdom, and the United States (see Exhibit 4.1). Or you can focus on the receiver of the message. For example, a smoking cessation clinic states, "We know you're trying to stop smoking. We think we can help."

Exhibit 4.1. Warning Label on a Cigarette Package.

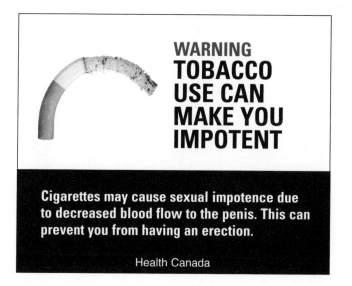

Frames

We rely on more than just words to take in information, interpret it, and make decisions. One of the most practical insights into how people make meaning is frame theory or strategic frame analysis. Frames are internalized mental ordering systems that allow us to chunk information meaningfully (Lakoff & Johnson, 1979; Lakoff, 2004). Frames also exist in the messages themselves. (Other terms used to refer to this mental chunking are *scripts* and *narrative*.) It would be very difficult for us to take in information unless we had a framework to fit it into.

A Frame at Work

Read this sentence:

"John came to school as usual today." What do you surmise about John?

Now read this second sentence:

"And when he got here the principal asked him to teach an extra class." Now what do you surmise about John?

Frames are powerful, often unconscious understandings that affect how and what information we select and how we understand that information. Take the example of a diabetic patient speaking with a health educator. The health educator is discussing the importance of following a diabetes management plan where food consumption, blood level testing, and activities of daily living are accounted for. Over time, it is clear that the patient is not complying with the regimen or sticking to the plan. The provider and the patient most likely have very different frames for understanding this management plan. The health educator may frame disease as a knowable enemy, one that can be defeated. The patient's frame for disease may be that it is fated and part of growing older: it will take its course one way or another.

Along with frames for organizing information, narratives or story structures are essential tools people use for comprehending information (Propp, 1968; van Dijk, 1977; Schank & Abelson, 1977). For example, read the following two sentences:

A Very Short Story
The King died.
The Queen died.

We read these two sentences as essentially isolated pieces of information. Now with one small change in the wording, something large happens to our understanding:

The King died.
Then the Queen died of grief.

We read the second example more like a "story" with a time frame and characters acting causally. These are two vital elements that story lines add to the scaffolding in order for messages to cohere and have more meaning. We use frames and narratives to process information and we do this quickly and automatically based on our skills and abilities.

When the reader can discern the frame of a message, this often helps to comprehend the message. For instance, when reading an information text a reader looks for the most important message. However, when a reader reads a story, she or he gets ready to attend to characters, their actions, and their states of being. There is often a beginning, middle, and end or resolution. However, if the language of the text does not make the type of text or frame obvious, readers are put at a disadvantage and have to work harder to make meaning, leaving much more room for misreading. This is especially true for less literate readers. (A good example of using a cultural frame to instruct about diabetes is found in Chapter 12, the case history of the Lakota Plains Indian health model.)

The bottom line is that effective communication is the sum total of many components, and much of what gets communicated is not only in the message (the content) but also in the context, codes, channels, and frames. This is an essential concept that can be put to use by those developing public health communications. (See the guidelines in Chapter 14.)

Meaning Making

People are essentially meaning makers when it comes to language. To a greater or lesser degree, depending on our abilities, we are also able to make ambiguous language clear. Read the following ambiguous simple sentence (which draws on a classic Noam Chomsky example): "Waking dragons can be dangerous." Depending on the context, we can understand this message as that if you wake a dragon, you may be in danger, or that a dragon, waking up, can be dangerous. If the text were, "Waking dragons can be dangerous. I wouldn't advise doing it even when you're feeling particularly courageous," the intended meaning becomes clearer.

We understand and use spoken and written language in a number of ways:

- Language is symbolic. We know that the word *medicine* is not the actual thing but stands for the thing.

- We generally understand more than we can produce.

- We perceive some spoken language as action (speech acts). For example, saying, "I apologize" or "I promise," actually performs acts as they are spoken, and "This foot hurts more than ever," spoken by a patient to the doctor, is understood by the doctor as a request for help.

- When we encounter hard-to-understand language, we skip over or guess about the meaning of an unknown

word. As we accumulate more context we can make
better guesses about the word's meaning.

- We use experience and context to understand what we
  read, hear, and see.

Reading

Often there is a critical mismatch between complex written and spoken health information and abilities to understand it. Far too many
health messages and materials are written at the 10- to 12-grade level
and higher. Web-based information presents even greater challenges
to the reader. When we add to this the language and jargon of science, medicine, and the health care system, many people lack sufficient health literacy to stay well. The versatility and power inherent
in the many forms language can take are often not put to work in
health communication and education. The language becomes rigid,
and it taxes the weaknesses of language users rather than capitalizing on their strengths.

As discussed in Chapter 3, the dominant approach to tackling
the issues of low health literacy in the public has been to simplify
messages. There is no denying that simpler language, less complex
vocabulary, jettisoning jargon, and surgically removing cumbersome
sentences improves comprehension. But there is a catch or two.
One is that you can find complexity in the strangest places.

Florida's ballot for the 2000 presidential election, shown in
Exhibit 4.2, was plagued with design problems that made reading
and using this document questionable. Voters had a hard time knowing what punch hole went with what candidate. Producers of print
information, and health information in general, are often so competent with the content that they find it easy to assume that receivers have the same competency. The result is that the messages
they create for the intended audiences do not always work.

A second catch is that we can make meaning out of the strangest
things. Read the following message from an e-mail widely circulated

Exhibit 4.2. 2000 Florida Presidential Election Ballot.

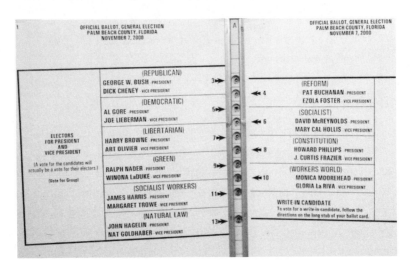

on the internet in the fall of 2003 (Davis, 2003): "Aoccdrnig to a rscheearch at Cmabrigde Uinervtisy, it deosn't mttaer in waht oredr the ltteers in a wrod are, the olny iprmoetnt tihng is taht the frist and lsat ltteer be at the rghit pclae. The rset can be a total mses and you can sitll raed it wouthit a porbelm. Tihs is bcuseae the huamn mnid deos not raed ervey lteter by istlef, but the wrod as a wlohe." Quite amazing, wouldn't you say?

With a little head scratching, you probably were able to read this (and might have gotten a chuckle out of your surprising skill as well!). When a text is hard to read, readers generally persist, rearranging the text to make some meaning, even if it is not the text's intended meaning. This is not true of extremely low-literate readers (third grade and lower) who are overwhelmed by any amount of print. While it is far beyond the scope of this book to discuss the many complex skills involved in reading, keep this e-mail teaser in mind as we discuss health messages in the case studies in later chapters.

As the scaffolding model of communication in Table 4.1 depicts, our skills and competencies for comprehending language vary based on whether we are reading, listening, or viewing. Four basic characteristics of print information determine the complexity of written text and also hold true for spoken language, with some variations, which will be discussed:

- Vocabulary

- Sentences

- Cohesion

- Relevance and context

(Beyond the scope of this book is a discussion of the wealth of reading research identifying other important skills such as metacognitive skills—knowing the function of reading a particular text, gauging importance, perceiving text structure—as well as strategies for fix-up and study strategies, and self-monitoring strategies. See Orasanu, 1986, for a good overview of reading.)

Vocabulary

Experts in any field develop and use language that is specific to that field and their work. Car mechanics talk about "torque" and "suspension," environmentalists refer to "sustainability" and "stewardship," physicians speak about "inflammatory conditions" and "chemotherapy protocols," public health officials discuss "relative risk," and health regulators and insurers talk about "eligibility" and "verification." Simplifying vocabulary (including idiosyncratic jargon) is critical in order to improve consumer/patient understanding of health information and advance health literacy. Here are some typical examples of simplifying vocabulary:

Term	Simplification
contagious	can get, catch
inoculations	shots
exacerbate	make it worse
prudent	careful, cautious
premium	what you pay

Sentences

There are essentially three important aspects of sentences that have strong implications for how they should be constructed for clarity.

- Sentence length

- Sentence complexity: grammar, sentence structure, and syntax

- Sentence cohesion: connection between sentences and between paragraphs

Exhibit 4.3 presents some truths about sentence complexity. One of them is that length alone does not make a sentence hard to read or listen to. Long sentences can be simple when they use the simple conjunctions *or, and,* or *but.* Phrases and clauses relate one clause to another and subordinate information as well. When the main noun and verb are distant from each other (for example, interrupted by clauses), the sentence becomes more complex and is therefore harder to read and listen to. Consider this sentence: "The virus, which has now been found to be antibiotic resistant, is going to be hard to treat." The information that the sentence is actually about—being resistant to antibiotics—is found in a clause, and reading clauses requires higher-level reading abilities. (Comprehending this sentence in spoken language would be affected by phrasing and emphasis.)

Exhibit 4.3. Three Sentence Truths.

Shorter is not always better:
Flying planes can be dangerous.

Longer is not always harder:
The mouse ate the cheese and the cake and the apple and
the cookies and the ice cream.

But hard is hard:
The boy who chased the cat that the dog barked at cried.

A complex sentence can become easier to read when there are simple sentences around it that repeat or reinforce the information. In the following example, the complex (and fairly improbable) sentence in italics is more likely to be negotiated by a reader because the surrounding information allows the reader to deduce who could be crying:

The boy was always afraid of dogs—especially barking dogs. One day he decided to chase a cat down the street. That's when he saw the big dog. The dog was on the porch and was looking at him and the cat. Then, it happened. The dog started barking real loud. *The boy, who chased the cat that the dog barked at, cried.* And when he got home, his mother said, "Next time you probably shouldn't go chasing cats. This way the dog won't bark and frighten you."

Cohesion

One unintended but common negative by-product of simplifying health messages (often print material) is that the message can actually become more difficult to read or listen to. This by-product usually occurs when all the cohesion is simplified (deleted) away. *Cohesion* refers to the ties that keep sentences and paragraphs connected and referring to each other (Halliday & Hasan, 1976).

When we hear or read a passage of text that is more than one sentence in length, we "usually can tell if it is a unified whole or just a list of sentences" (Halliday & Hasan, 1976, p. 2). To understand most messages (texts), another element in the text, referred to as the *tie*, must be used. The text is created when the interpretation of one element is dependent on another. Halliday and Hasan (1976) use a simple example of the principle of cohesion: "Wash and core six cooking apples. Put them into a fireproof dish." *Them* is dependent on a tie made to the apples in the earlier sentence. Much evidence from reading research has demonstrated that reading and listening comprehension are greatly influenced by the level and type of cohesion in a text or other message. Texts with little or no cohesion are harder to read, understand, and remember (Mandler & Johnson, 1977; Kintsch, Kozminsky, Streby, McKoon, & Keenan, 1975; Kintsch, 1977; van Dijk, 1977).

Cohesion is critical to comprehension, and yet often it is not present in health messages. In the example in Exhibit 4.4, the health message (text) on the left lacks simple cohesion. The reader has to work hard at making the inferences by filling in the blanks. What is folic acid? Why would I take a multivitamin (a difficult word) if I need "acid"? What is the relationship between folic acid and birth defects of the spine and brain? The sentence on the right is clearer because it uses cohesion: there are more obvious ties between sentences. Preserving cohesion creates a logical flow between and across sentences and utterances, and readers rely on this. Chapter 14 provides a number of examples of how to use cohesion to evaluate material and compose material for greater comprehension.

Relevance and Context

People use context to interpret messages all the time. The context can include things such as life experience, knowledge base, and mental frames. The following example demonstrates how important context is for reading comprehension. It was used in a classic reading study in 1972 (Bransford & Johnson, 1972, p. 720), and still holds true today.

The procedure is actually quite simple. First you arrange the items in different groups. Of course one pile may be sufficient depending on how much there is to do. If you have to go somewhere else due to lack of facilities that is the next step; otherwise you are pretty well set.

What activity is this paragraph describing? If you're confused, you're not alone. But if you add a title to the text, "Washing Clothes," the paragraph makes much more sense. The title gives the reader a context, and that context gives the words and sentences meaning, precisely what reading researchers found in a controlled study of such passages. In a study assessing the ability of Medicaid and State Children's Health Insurance Plan (SCHIP) recipients to read and understand state notices regarding eligibility, we found that simplifying the language to provide context greatly improved the readability of complex language (Zarcadoolas et al., 2004).

Exhibit 4.4. Example of Cohesion.

Eat a healthy breakfast, lunch, and dinner every day, including green leafy vegetables, beans, citrus fruits and juices, and whole grain foods that contain folic acid. But remember, even healthy meals may not contain enough folic acid. Take a multivitamin each day to reduce the risk of birth defects of the spine and brain.	Eat healthy at least three times a day—breakfast, lunch, and dinner. Make sure you eat plenty of fruits and vegetables and whole grain cereals. And be sure to take a vitamin for pregnant women every day (a multivitamin). The food and the vitamin will give you folic acid. Folic acid helps prevent birth defects of the spine and brain. Even if you eat well every day, you should take a multivitamin with folic acid every day.

Spoken Language

Spoken language is the first step for most people on the road to becoming literate. Talk is fundamental to being literate, and much of what we learn about health comes from spoken, "through-the-air" communication: doctor-patient conversation, TV, radio, conversations with family and friends. Yet there is little research on the relationship of fundamental literacy, health literacy, and people's particular abilities to speak and listen meaningfully.

Talk Is Like a Ball Game

To better understand the power of spoken language it is a good idea to know some basics about how it functions. The linguist Charles Fillmore (1974) used the analogy of a game of catch to describe a spoken conversation. A person throws a ball to another person. That person catches the ball. Rather than put that ball down, pick up a new ball, and throw it, the catcher keeps the ball in play. When conversations are going well, the speaker and listener keep the ball in play.

Here is what it sounds like when the ball game does not go right:

> DOCTOR: Well, hello, Ms. James.
> MS. JAMES: Hello, Doctor. I really don't think the medicine we tried is working.
> DOCTOR: So, first, tell me—how are your grandkids?

Speakers rely on many subtle and not-so-subtle cues to interpret what is going on and to continue the conversation. Four key cues are the words, tone, gestures, and context. To see how speech intonation conveys meaning, read the following exchange aloud:

> TRAVELER: I'm going to California.
> QUESTIONER: Where?
> TRAVELER: Disney World.

Now read the exchange again, changing the intonation of *where*:

> TRAVELER: I'm going to California.
> QUESTIONER: (*With intonation of misunderstanding*) Where?
> TRAVELER: California.

In the first exchange *where* is spoken without a significant rising intonation. The traveler interprets this correctly as requiring more specific information. In the second exchange, *where* is spoken with a distinct rising intonation, signaling to the traveler that the message was not understood and needs to be repeated.

How skillfully one uses these cues will determine everything from how understandable each speaker is to who gets to hold the floor. In some situations, status or role determines who holds the floor. For example, a doctor speaking to a patient or a professor speaking to a class of students is likely to have the dominant conversational position. In other cases, verbal skill determines who holds the floor and who is more convincing. This is most apparent when we listen to two highly skilled speakers debating. We can find ourselves being swayed by one position and then the next, reminding us how powerful communication is.

Print Is More Than Speech Written Down

Probably the most important concept about spoken language and written language is that print is not simply speech written down, that is, transcription (Olson, 1977; Scribner & Cole, 1981; Tannen, 1982; Olson & Torrance, 2001). In many circumstances, what we say is really an action in a social situation, as in "Thank you" (thank), "Open the window" (request), and "Say thank you" (command) (Searle, 1969; Goffman, 1981). Spoken language often does not have as complicated a grammatical structure as print language, and it relies more on the immediate context of the speaker and listener. Grammatical complexity is not as much a barrier in spoken language as in written language because there is often an abundance of context to help the speakers understand each other. A speaker can talk to someone, pointing, using pronouns such as *this* or *that*, and using facial expressions and body language and intonation to carry much of the meaning (paralinguistic or nonverbal communication). The speaker and listener in conversations often rely on these paralinguistic cues to determine if both are following and understanding each other. In fact, the vast majority of what we communicate is carried in our nonverbal acts, not our words (Knapp & Hall, 2002). Speakers and listeners can monitor each other's understanding and adjust the conversation, using repetition, examples, familiar analogies, and many other linguistic devices to emphasize and clarify. These cues are not usually present in print.

Print language is more decontextualized than speech; the reader has to rely more on the words. Often the tone and form of written text are apparent and useful only for more skilled readers. Readers also use information such as who generated the message (for example, the government, their doctor, or some other trusted source) and what type of text the message is (a letter conveying a decision about health benefits, an information text about a medical condition, or a story about a patient or consumer in similar circumstances).

The following example demonstrates the important variation in the structure and function of spoken and written texts. We use an excerpt from a television interview about avian flu (2006) and print text about the topic from the Centers for Disease Control and Prevention (CDC) web site. As you read these two passages, note how the language varies and how you are interpreting the messages:

Television Interview with Infectious Disease Expert

DR. OSTERHOLM: Today in this world where we have so many poultry. In 1969, again, the last pandemic, China had 12 million chickens. . . . Today it has 15 *billion*. That's how much it's changed. We have an endless supply. . . .

OPRAH: Should we not be eating chickens?

DR. O: No. Chicken is a very good food, by the way. It's perfectly safe food in this country. I don't worry about chicken. I want . . . to make sure that Americans understand this. But the point is around the world, where these chickens are kept out in the open, where they're not protected by these secure barns, each one of those is in a sense a virus test tube. And we keep replenishing them because people need protein.

OPRAH: And who is it that's most at risk for contracting the bird flu?

DR. O: Over there it's the people having close contact with the infected chicken. But I worry about all these chickens where the mutations are going to occur. So one day the virus that you and I worry about here in the Midwest is actually a virus that finally had its final mutation—this kind of genetic roulette table was in China somewhere, was in Vietnam, was in Thailand— it may have been in Turkey. That's why, as much as this circulates [gesturing circle] today, in a sense, also we have the perfect setup for this virus to continue to mutate.

OPRAH: OK. So what should we be doing as a nation? What should the media be doing? Because what's going to happen, it mutates, you're going to have panic. People are just going to be panicked and crazy. [Winfrey, 2006]

The expert in this interview goes on to provide clear recommendations about what the government and people need to do to be better prepared. The discussion then continues as follows:

OPRAH: If I'm hearing you correctly, what I thought you said about the bird flu makes me very worried that we're not paying attention in the right way [questioning intonation].

DR. O: Of the priorities in the world that we have right now, which are many and are important, I can't imagine a more important one from the social, economic, political, health, or just moral basis than this. It is really *something*. It is going to happen. How bad it's going to be, we don't know. But it's not a guess, it is going to. And what we need to do is so much more to be better prepared for it.

OPRAH: And the bottom line is we're not prepared now?

DR. O: We as a world are hardly prepared at all. [Winfrey, 2006]

Meanwhile, the CDC offers these "Key Facts About Avian Influenza" on their web site.

Avian Influenza in Birds

Avian influenza is an infection caused by avian (bird) influenza (flu) viruses. These influenza viruses occur naturally among birds. Wild birds worldwide carry the viruses in their intestines, but usually do not get sick from them. However, avian influenza is very contagious among birds and can make some domesticated birds, including chickens, ducks, and turkeys, very sick and kill them.

Infected birds shed influenza virus in their saliva, nasal secretions, and feces. Susceptible birds become infected when they have contact with contaminated secretions or excretions or with surfaces that are contaminated with secretions or excretions from infected birds. Domesticated birds may become infected with avian influenza virus through direct contact with infected waterfowl or other infected poultry, or through contact with surfaces (such as dirt or cages) or materials (such as water or feed) that have been contaminated with the virus.

Infection with avian influenza viruses in domestic poultry causes two main forms of disease that are distinguished by low and high extremes of virulence. The "low pathogenic" form may go undetected and usually causes only mild symptoms (such as ruffled feathers and a drop in egg production). However, the highly pathogenic form spreads more rapidly through flocks of poultry. This form may cause disease that affects multiple internal organs and has a mortality rate that can reach 90 to 100 percent, often within forty-eight hours. [Centers for Disease Control and Prevention, 2006]

In the first example—the television interview (spoken language)—the two speakers actively try to collaborate to be understood and move the conversation along from topic to topic. The speaker and listener alternate roles, interrupt with questions, and easily move into short stories. Although the sentence structure varies from short phrases to long, rambling ones and the vocabulary is of varied difficulty, the participants are sensitive to what is being understood and what needs clarification through emphasis or repetition or use of analogies.

In contrast, the second example of print language relies heavily on sequential ordering of information. There is less context to help interpret complex vocabulary or syntax, and readers cannot rely on intonation as clues. There is little if any repetition and no clear markers telling the reader how to prioritize what is most important. This type of print can present real barriers for less fluent readers.

Acknowledging and using the similarities and differences in spoken and written communication are important in planning successful health promotion programs and specific health communication messages. In the examples about avian flu, some changes that would make the messages more understandable are using repetition in the spoken text and unpacking or simplifying the vocabulary and sentence structure of the print text. (See Chapters 5 and 14.)

Table 4.2 lists some of the differences in structure and function of spoken and written language.

Individuals with low literacy skills are often able to speak and understand oral language that is at least two grade levels above the level at which they read. This can be seen most dramatically in videotapes and transcripts of patients as they speak. In the following two passages, both of the individuals with low literacy are using spoken language that they are most likely not able to read with comprehension. For example, see the AMA video *Low Health Literacy: You Can't Tell by Looking* quoted below.

> I had an abscess in my ear one time [gesturing to ear]. Well, I had to fill out forms and I couldn't fill out. So I didn't go. I come back home. And I ended up having to go to the emergency room that night, because it burst [male patient, second-grade reading skills].

> Can you imagine what it's like, you being a patient and sick? And you know that you have limited skills and you're talking to an intelligent doctor, like yourself. Well, and these people are using words that you really don't know, because they're not speaking in laymen's terms. OK? Most doctors are just presuming that everybody's intelligent as they are. And that is just not the case. So, what you do, you come out of that room, that examination room, with this intelligent woman or man, thinking, God, I hope I don't make a mistake with my medicine because I didn't understand anything he said to me [female patient, third-grade reading level]. [American Medical Association Foundation, 2003]

**Table 4.2. Differences in Structure and
Function of Spoken and Written Language.**

Characteristics of Spoken Language	Characteristics of Written Language
Highly dependent on context	More decontextualized
Interaction focused two ways	Interaction focused one way
Message and intent focused	Message focused
Ephemeral, fleeting	Permanent, archival (can refer back to it)
Memory (mnemonics) needed	
Meaning more overt	Relies on record rather than memory
Cohesion carried in interactive cues—intonation, body language	Meaning subject to more interpretation
	Cohesion carried in reference words: "this," "he," "that doctor"

In these examples, the speakers use:

- Difficult vocabulary at approximately 8th- to 12th-grade level—for example, *abscess, emergency, burst, intelligent, examination, laymen's, presuming*

- Compound sentences—for example, connected with *and*

- Complex sentences using clauses and phrases—for example, "because it burst," "words that you really don't know," "because they're not speaking in laymen's terms"

- Cohesion across almost all their sentences by using appropriate pronouns and reference—for example, "it," "these people," connectors ("well," "so"), and rhetorical devices ("So, what do you do?" "Can you imagine?")

Implications for Spoken and Written Health Messages

Because print is not simply speech written down, there are opportunities for health professionals to capitalize on the different characteristics of each modality. Often patients and other consumers who have difficulty reading a message may be able to understand a spoken message better. Because of the load on auditory memory, these messages have to contain facilitators such as brevity, narrative structure, or repetition. Print or some other visual representations can then be used to reinforce the information. (See Chapter 14.)

There is an opportunity to use spoken language and print supportively. That people's spoken language abilities often exceed their reading and writing skills has implications for capitalizing on spoken language skills to enhance health promotion and communication strategies. However, greater fluency with spoken language is a doubled-edged sword in health promotion. It makes sense that low-literate individuals are likely to rely disproportionately on spoken information (television, radio, conversation) and not be able to substantiate or corroborate that information. (See Chapter 5.) This unfortunately can become a self-fulfilling action as low-literate individuals continue to use channels that do not improve their literacy. (For guidelines for capitalizing on spoken language skills, see Chapter 14.)

Many generic health campaigns are driven by the tacit assumption that one size fits all. Top-down models of health promotion and communication are often generic and aimed at the broadest audience. However, there is ample evidence that collaborative efforts of health promotion, informed by the needs and desires of specific target audiences, are likely to have greater impact on health status (McKenzie-

Mohr & Smith, 1999; Dela, Chim, & Jenkins, 1998; Berkowitz, 2000; Roussos & Fawcett, 2000; Institute of Medicine, 2003).

There is a tremendously wide range of ways that people can and do use language to read, listen, and view messages. Therefore, knowing about the target audience is central to effective health communication. Spoken language abilities, reading skills, sense of self, relevancy of the topic, and those people trust for information are just a few of the vitally important elements that can make or break health promotion efforts. Using qualitative and ethnographic methods to learn from and collaborate with your intended audience are ways to ensure you are developing the right messages at the right time. (See the guidelines in Chapter 14 for further discussion.)

Wrapping Up

In this chapter, we have argued that to be truly successful in health promotion, education, and communication, and to advance the public's health literacy, we need to understand the power and flexibility of dynamic language in use. And while language and literacy skills vary greatly in people, we can make a more deliberate effort to capitalize on what people can do rather than tax the very skills they are lacking.

Exercises

1. Collect and examine print health materials. List the specific types of complexity that would present obstacles to average readers. Rewrite some of these examples for improved readability using strategies on the vocabulary, sentence structure, and cohesion levels.

2. Compare a television message for a popular pharmaceutical with print material addressing the same type of medication

produced by a traditional health information source—for example, a health foundation or health department. List the vocabulary, sentence structure, and cohesion characteristics of these two different messages and what these characteristics demand of the reader, listener, or viewer. What strategies does the television message use? Are any of these strategies transferable to print?

3. Using a videotape of a patient or consumer, note the differences between the form and structures of the language they are speaking versus their ability to read. If you do not have access to such a video, we recommend *Health Literacy: You Can't Tell by Looking* (American Medical Association Foundation, 2003).

5

The Traditional Mass Media

Are we too fat, too thin, too old, or is our hair too gray? Are our memories failing, our sex lives lagging? Do we eat correctly, exercise enough, and use the best type of toothpaste? If we are not sure about the answers to those questions and a host of others, we can simply change the television channel, and there is sure to be an advertisement, a news broadcast, or an entertainment program telling us what we should or should not do and whom we should aspire to be like.

The mass media present both complex and overly simplistic messages about health. They can improve health literacy, or reduce health literacy. The mass media can positively and negatively influence the activity level, worldview, and dietary habits of their audiences. Mass media can educate individuals about healthy behavior, or establish powerful role models for harmful behavior. Thus, for health practitioners and communicators concerned about improving health through improving health literacy, a basic familiarity and understanding of the mass media is an absolute must. That is the central task of this chapter.

This chapter addresses how the mass media operate and introduces the health literacy skills required to interpret media content. In particular, the issues highlighted in this chapter relate to the domain of civic literacy. We begin with an introduction to several traditional media. Then we discuss key types of media content:

entertainment, news, and advertising. The chapter closes with a brief description of tools for health communicators. Chapter 6 discusses the newest mass medium, the internet.

Introduction to Mass Media

Even in the early days of the mass media, the issues of the role of the press in society and the tension between news and advertising content were quite apparent. Perhaps the most frequently quoted words about the role of the press as a watchdog of government come from Thomas Jefferson: "Were it left to me to decide whether we should have a government without newspapers, or newspapers without a government, I should not hesitate for a moment to prefer the latter." However, in notable contrast to that ideal view of media content, the third president of the United States also wrote, "Advertisements contain the only truths to be relied on in a newspaper."

The sheer magnitude of the choices available argues for efforts to enhance the skills of individuals to understand, interpret, and judge the relevance and truthfulness of advertising, entertainment, and news in the mass media. Both praise and criticism abound in the academic literature that looks at connections between the mass media and health—for example:

- A Nielsen Media Research study found children and adolescents in the United States watch nearly three hours of television per day, not including video games or videotapes. On average, estimates are that a television is turned on in American households around seven hours per day.

- The mass media are home to over $2 billion of efforts to market pharmaceuticals directly to the public, a phenomenon with both positive and negative outcomes (Gollust, Hull, & Wilfond, 2002).

- The mass media fuel an ongoing fear of germs. They build this fear by developing the theme of the "revenge of the superbugs" (Tomes, 2000).

- Mass media campaigns have, to varying magnitudes, been associated with declines in smoking rates (Levy & Friend, 2000).

- Multiple studies indicate a relationship between the amount of television watched and perceptions of one's own body, as well as symptoms of eating disorders (Botta, 1999; Committee on Public Education, 2001; Harrison & Cantor, 1997; Posovac, Posovac, & Posovac, 1998; Stice & Shaw, 1994).

- The average young TV viewer in the United States is exposed to more than 14,000 sexual references each year, only a few of which portray responsible sexual behavior or accurate information about birth control, abstinence, or the risks of pregnancy and sexually transmitted diseases (Committee on Public Education, 1999).

- Mass media, mass education, and mass consumerism are placing new demands on the medical community and increasing the demands and knowledge of patients (Neuberger, 2000).

The mass media exist due to a combination of technology and social structure. The emergence and growth of the mass media would not have been possible without technological inventions including photography, videotape, the telegraph, and telephone, the printing press, the television, and now the internet. Socially, the mass media require a literate society because literacy creates a demand for a wide range of information. Also, the mass media benefit from an urban society, as urban dwellers tend to need new sources of information and social connections to replace the personal contacts generally relied on in rural settings (DeFleur & Dennis, 2002). In the following sections, we briefly identify and discuss several of the traditionally dominant mass media.

Newspapers

With the exception of books, newspapers are the oldest of today's major mass media. At the broadest level, newspapers can be roughly defined as publications that are:

- Published at least weekly

- Produced on paper by a mechanical printing process or delivered online

- Available to people of all walks of life

- Of general interest

- Readable by people of ordinary literacy

- Timely

- Stable over time

A first aspect of newspaper content is the way it is categorized. Newspapers divide content into sections, the most common of which are news, business, living/lifestyle, opinion/editorial, business, and sports. As newspapers grow larger, the number and variety of sections increase.

A second aspect of newspaper content is its reliance on written text and still photographs. Unlike radio, a newspaper cannot employ sound as a tool, and unlike television or the internet, a newspaper cannot rely on moving images. Those inherent characteristics directly influence the way information can be packaged and is received by the readers.

Newspaper Readership

- On average, 65.1 percent of those polled report reading newspapers daily or regularly (Pew Research Center, 2001a).

- Newspaper readership increases with age: 74.1 percent of those 65 years and older but only 51.9 percent of those 18 to 24 years old reported reading a newspaper daily or regularly (Pew Research Center, 2001a).

- Men and women report reading newspapers with generally the same frequency (General Social Survey, 2000).

- Newspaper readership levels rise as income levels rise. For example, around 71 percent of those with incomes over $20,000 report reading newspapers daily, whereas just over 56 percent of individuals with an income under $19,999 report doing so (General Social Survey, 2000).

- Newspaper readership varies dramatically by race; for example, 40 percent of white respondents reported reading newspapers daily, while only 26.9 percent of black respondents reported doing so (General Social Survey, 2000).

An important third aspect of newspaper content for those wishing to communicate successfully about health and improve health literacy is the distinction between news, opinion, and advertising, as all are used in health education and communication campaigns. Newspapers in particular, and the news-gathering media in general, purport to maintain a clean line between news, opinion, and advertising. *News* refers in general to the content produced by journalists. *Opinion* refers to the content on the editorial/opinion page and includes the newspaper's editorial, op-eds, political and editorial cartoons, and letters to the editor. *Advertising* refers to paid content, generally promoting the goods and services of a business, individual, or organization.

Who Follows Health News?

Women report following health news more closely than men: 64.9 percent of men report following health news very or somewhat closely, whereas 78.9 percent of women reported doing so (Pew Research Center, 2001a).

People between 55 and 64 years of age report following health news the most, with 83.9 percent of the people in that age group reporting doing so very or somewhat closely. People 18 to 24 years of age are the least likely, with 52.8 percent of that age group doing so (Pew Research Center, 2001a).

However, the line between news, opinion, and advertising is frequently stretched and often broken, creating a challenge to the audience, particular those with low health literacy skills, to discern among them. For instance, media outlets often allow, for a price of course, advertisers to place their advertisements next to news content related to their product. During early 2004, many television stations aired news video releases prepared by the Bush administration to promote its Medicare prescription drug plan without identifying the government as the producer, an action that the U.S. Government Accountability Office (2004) called an illegal use of taxpayers' dollars.

Magazines

Especially since the debut of television, the focus of magazines has shifted from large circulation, general interest publications, like *Life* or *Look,* to magazines targeting special interest readerships, like *Car and Driver* and *Self.*

Numerous magazines focus on health, medicine, and fitness. Magazines aimed specifically at medical practitioners are classified as trade magazines, while magazines such as *Fitness* are considered consumer magazines. In 2002, the largest circulation magazine with a health focus was *Medizine,* which was also the fastest-growing magazine in 1997 and 1998. According to *AdAge, Medizine* was the 13th largest magazine by circulation in the United States in 2002. *Modern Maturity* had the largest circulation, *Readers Digest* second, and *TV Guide* third. Other magazines with a focus on health and self-help in the top 300 circulation magazines, with their ranking in parentheses, are *Men's Health* (43), *Shape* (46), *Health* (62), *Fitness* (68), *Weight Watchers* (119), *Men's Fitness* (138), *Fit Pregnancy in Español* (170), *Fit Pregnancy* (171), and *Muscle and Fitness* (199) (AdAge.com, 2002).

Books

Books have the longest production time of the mass media. They can take anywhere from a decade, in a few cases, to a matter of months to write and publish. Books are also the oldest of the mass media.

Unlike the other mass media, books are generally not supported by advertising revenue but survive on sales to readers alone. The medium is generally considered a higher-quality venue for publishing than either magazines or newspapers. The length and the ability of books to present greater complexity raise the hurdles to readers, making books in general the most challenging for readers with lower literacy levels. Nevertheless, books can be successfully written for readers at all literacy levels.

Radio

Radio used to be the dominant medium in the United States and remains so in much of the rest of the world. In the United States, some cherish the so-called golden age of radio when families sat together around the living room radio listening to the next installment of popular radio dramas and comedies such as *The Shadow* or *Fibber McGee and Molly*. Since the advent of television, radio, like magazines, has made efforts to target specific audiences by changes in format and content rather than try to appeal to everyone all the time. Types of radio content vary from talk to music and in different languages. There are radio stations broadcasting in Spanish and Native American languages and radio stations that feature programs in a variety of languages including Greek, Irish, Chinese, and Japanese.

As a medium, radio is limited to transmitting sound. Unlike the printed mass media, reading skills are not required to understand radio content, and unlike newspapers, books, television, and films, radio content cannot include still or moving images. Therefore, the listener employs a range of skills to decode the spoken language without the help of written text or visuals. That limitation places special demands on storytellers, journalists, and advertisers to create narratives with dramatic elements to engage the listener, but it can lower the threshold for listeners because written literacy skills are not required. Therefore, complex messages, which are generally more difficult to convey, understand, and remember, are not served well by radio.

A successful media strategy employing radio is to design campaigns that reinforce radio messages with print and visual messages in other mass media. These efforts have an advantage in terms of exposure, recognition, comprehension, and impact. In the health care arena, pharmaceutical companies often skillfully use this strategy in promoting specific drugs or conditions.

For health communicators, radio is generally an effective and affordable way to get information out quickly and to specific audiences. Radio can serve as an effective element in a mix of media to announce upcoming events or news of general interest, as well to deliver health notices and updates to specific audiences when necessary. Internationally, radio is one of the most effective forms of mass media since television has not gained the saturation worldwide that it has in the United Sates. A study by the Joint United Nations Programme on HIV/AIDS (UNAIDs), for instance, found that radio was one of the most effective media across Africa to convey information aimed at educating individuals about how to prevent and respond to the threat of HIV/AIDs.

Television

Among the mass media, television is the 900-pound gorilla in the living room everyone is talking about. In the United States, 83 percent of the 2,636 respondents to the Centers for Disease Control's 1999 Healthstyles survey (1999) said they most often learned something about diseases or how to prevent them from television. Newspapers and magazines were the next most used sources at 78 percent; a combination of family friends, doctors, nurses, and others were used by 71 percent; radio by 24 percent; the internet by 13 percent; and hot lines by only 1 percent of the respondents to the survey. Twenty percent of those responding agreed that they have difficulty understanding a lot of the health information they read, and 13 percent agreed they never seem to find good answers to their health questions and concerns.

On average, people spend more time watching television than they do with any of the other mass media. They also spend more time watching television than most other activities in their lives.

Today nearly every household in the United States has at least one television set, and a majority of households have more than one. The pervasiveness of television in daily life is the main source of

---

Television Viewers

- African American households and Hispanic households both spend more time watching television than the average viewer in the United States. That is true across all age groups as well as through the daytime, prime time, and late night viewing slots (http://www.nielsonmedia.com/ethnicmeasure).

- People aged 65 and older are nearly twice as likely as those under age 30 to have watched news on television (Pew Research Center, 2001a).

---

the power television has (Shanahan & Morgan, 1999). Perhaps the easiest way to understand the power of television is to imagine life in the United States without it. Without television, millions would not be able to watch the SuperBowl every year, millions would not have been able to watch O. J. Simpson try to put on the gloves, there would likely not be a World Wrestling Federation, we would not know within minutes that a major earthquake struck somewhere in the world, and reality TV shows would have never been made. Many Americans might never have heard what passes for medical discourse on televisions shows like *MASH* and *ER*.

Television presents a mix of words and moving pictures in an effective and enchanting combination. That marriage of words and pictures draws individuals in through its ability to present messages on multiple levels simultaneously. That, in effect, lowers the burden on the viewer, making television an easy medium to spend time with. Consider how many times in your own life, perhaps each day, the flickering image of a television screen has caught your attention and drawn you in.

The bulk of television content is advertising, and a growing number of the messages about health are in the form of direct-to-consumer (DTC) advertising of pharmaceuticals. Many, if not most, of the messages Americans receive about health come from television and the majority of those messages promote commercial products.

Advertising is not the only source of health information on television. When viewers turn to television news, a significant amount of what they watch is directed at health issues. According to data collected annually by the Center for Media and Public Affairs, health issues were the third most discussed topic on the nightly news through the 1990s. That does not include the plethora of so-called news magazine programs like *60 Minutes* or *Dateline* where content is not as driven by daily events so that health is likely even a higher percentage of the overall content.

Television clearly plays a significant role in terms of delivering health information to Americans. Furthermore, it helps set the stage for all information about health and health-related behavior that individuals encounter in their daily lives from all sources.

Media Content: Challenges and Opportunities to Advance Health Literacy

In this section, we briefly outline three main types of mass media content that frequently contain health information: entertainment, news, and advertising. Receivers of mass media messages, however, do not always make the same distinctions. Thus, some argue that the aggregate media exposure across content and different media is the source of the strongest effect.

Entertainment

Health, medicine, and science allow storytellers in the media to address the promise of the unknown, portray a human ability to overcome that unknown, and depict threats that arise from nature.

As a result, there is a long history of television drama, films, and novels that focus on issues of health and medicine, including everything from the emergency room focus of the television drama *ER* to *The Andromeda Strain*, a classic science-fiction book and then a film, featuring a killer microbe.

There is great potential for delivering positive health messages through entertainment. As one of the largest shared activities of Americans, entertainment programs can reach many people with identical messages at the same time. Entertainment programming is engaging in a way that news programs and documentaries are generally not, so educational lessons can be included without the barriers encountered in traditional education settings.

For example, in 1989, a network television show, *Who's the Boss*, delivered a message about underage drinking that was part of a campaign by the Harvard School of Public Health. Such efforts seem to be even more common internationally, as entertainment-oriented television programs addressing public health issues have been created in many countries, including South Africa, India, Cuba, and Pakistan.

One concern is that depictions of health care in entertainment programming do not always reflect reality. For instance, there is very little waiting for a doctor on television, and there are generally plenty of nurses, medications, and life-saving surgeries available, especially at the last minute. On American television, doctors and nurses are outnumbered only by criminals and law enforcement personnel. In addition, almost everyone recovers to full health in entertainment programming, even from serious diseases requiring heroic measures by doctors (Signorelli, 1990).

Another concern about entertainment programming relates to the depiction of actions that can lead to negative health outcomes, such as violence and the use of alcohol and cigarettes. The average American child watches 8,000 murders and 100,000 other assorted acts of violence before finishing elementary school. There are a large number of references to cigarettes, alcohol, and illicit drugs on television. For example, one-fourth of MTV videos were found to contain alcohol or tobacco use (Committee on Public Education, 2001).

News

The news is determined through a selection process involving a number of actors from journalists and editors to information sources such as scientists, doctors, politicians, civil servants, and organizations of all types. In addition, individuals select what is news to them from the range of news presented. Thus, news is a social construction that reflects the social setting, needs, and values of the participants.

The civic domain of health literacy inherently involves the skills needed to understand some of the basic forces that construct the news agenda and an ability to interpret the mixed messages and competing meanings often encountered in the news.

There are many competing definitions of news. Some take a simple approach and assert that news is what interests people. A little thought about the process of news gathering quickly expands that approach to a perhaps more realistic notion that news is what news editors and journalists think will interest people. That definition, however, gives way to the need for analytical categories through which the news can be studied and better understood.

A leading communication researcher, Kathleen Hall Jamieson, argues that hard news can be relatively well identified by the following attributes (Jamieson & Campbell, 1997):

- A dramatic action or event

- Quickly identified and understood

- About people

- About an issue people care about or can be convinced to care about

- Novel, deviant, or out of the ordinary

- Reports events linked to issues prevalent in the news at the time

The inverse of those news values is partially summed up by an example of a news headline American audiences will very likely never see: "Small Storm Last Week in Nigeria Hurts No One."

No matter how important something may be to health professionals, if it does not have at least some news value, it is not likely to be included in the news. Table 5.1 shows the many areas of

Table 5.1. Areas of Potential Mismatch.

News Values	Public Health Campaigns
Reflect society	Change society
Personalize	Aggregate/generalize
Cover short-term events	Create long-term campaigns
Magnitude—bigger is better	Often specific groups are at risk
Proximity—closer is better	Can be diffuse and widespread or focused on small, specific populations or places
Timeliness—newer is better	Often take time to develop
Frequent—needs news every day	Often not predictable
Surprising—draws attention	Surprises are bad
Competitive—scoop the competition	Want everyone to know
Clarity—easier is better	Often technically complex
Facts—science and facts are valued	Often scrambling for data
Popularity—well-known sources and subjects are better	Often focus on specific, at times marginalized, at-risk populations
Elitism—all experts are equally valued	Experts can disagree

potential conflict between the values that news-gathering organizations use in selecting and shaping the content of the news and the values of public health and health communication and promotion efforts (Anderson, 1997; Atkin, 1982; Bell, 1991).

An awareness of news values is clearly useful when shaping information to feed into the news production process as well as when interpreting news content. Health communicators will experience more success if they are able to shape their suggestions with these news values in mind.

Health and Science News

Everyone has some interest in how to maintain their own and their family's health, making news coverage of health both relevant and personal. Coverage of health issues can focus on practical, easy-to-read, how-to advice, fads and popular culture, or unexpected surprises. One estimate is that at least one out of every four articles in newspapers is health related (Wallack, 1990).

Health research is often presented as making "sudden breakthroughs," and recovery from serious illness can be touted as "miraculous." Such persuasive presentations in the news media often convince individuals that the reality of health and health care is vastly different than it actually is, where research is a slow, cumulative process and recovery from illness is more often the result of patient, dedicated, caregiving by trained professionals.

The contradictory nature of medical information as presented in the news is often confusing as well. For example, the efficacy of mammograms in battling breast cancer and prolonging life is, on one hand, denied by a single scientific study that makes headlines, while on the other hand, the news has consistently discussed regular mammography as an important procedure for the detection and cure of breast cancer. Or scientific "experts" have alternately appeared in the mass media promoting various vitamin and food supplements as enhancing and then later as detrimental to health.

A further area of concern in the reporting of health and science news is related to the use of sources of information and the agendas they may bring to the news. One central health literacy skill is the ability to decipher the presence of agendas in news coverage of health issues. Consumers of medical information should be aware, and informed, that the news can be presented in ways that deceive, for example, by self-interested or biased "authorities." The motivations of some information sources may be less apparent than the fairly obvious intent of advertising. For example, politicians and government officials may spin the information they provide to reassure their constituents and demonstrate that they are in control of the problem at hand.

The flow of information to a media outlet, particularly from official government sources, is in essence a subsidy provided to the press. Government officials and agencies routinely prepare and distribute information they want to see in the mass media, thereby lowering the costs of news-gathering. Hospitals, universities, and the range of institutions involved in health care and health research often employ staffs specifically for this function. Maintaining positive relationships with such sources of information can result in journalists and media organizations choosing to publish information that the sources desire to see distributed, or not publishing information the sources do not want made public even if it may be newsworthy.

An example of an agreement that affects the timing of health-related information distributed through the mass media is the practice of embargoing stories released by the major science publications such as *Science, Nature, JAMA,* and the *New England Journal of Medicine*. In return for advance notice of research reports so that journalists can have the time to prepare their articles, journalists agree not to publish until the scientific research article appears in the peer-reviewed academic journal. Thus, readers and viewers see announcements of new health research discoveries in a sudden onslaught, though the research has been ongoing for months or years. If journalists violate the embargo, they will no longer receive advance notice from the scientific journals. This practice is quite common and contributes to a popular misconception of health research consisting of a string of "Eureka!" moments for individuals rather than a slow accumulation of successes and failures by a community of researchers.

Dueling Experts

An unfortunately common journalistic strategy is the assumption that a balanced story is one that presents two sides to an issue. However, with complex issues such as those involved in health, there are rarely only two sides to an issue. In these instances, journalists should attempt to provide equal coverage to all sides of a complex issue rather than present two conflicting opinions of experts, but this would often leave the layperson confused, perhaps dismissing the experts because of the apparently contradictory information. However, mass media content is also received over time, and larger narratives can emerge that tell a different story about the incremental progress of scientific research, explaining apparent contradictions as new knowledge evolves. In addition, individuals often fill in the gaps between individual stories with knowledge already possessed (Seale, 2002). Ideally, health literacy skills would be strengthened to the point that individuals are aware of these issues as they peruse mass media content.

For example, following a recent spike in media coverage on the effects of certain types of hormonal replacement therapy (HRT) caused by release of a study reporting that the risks outweighed the benefits for women on combined estrogen-plus-progestin HRT, one survey found that every woman in the survey sample knew of the study. Half of the women reported making some change in their HRT as a result. However, half of the women who reported using estrogen alone changed their therapy, suggesting they did not completely understand the study's results as an important distinction between combination therapy and therapy with estrogen alone, which was underreported or missing altogether in many mass media reports (McIntosh & Blalock, 2005).

Advertising

Advertising is the engine and audiences are the fuel that run the mass media machine because advertising rates are generally based on audience size and type. Advertising has been present in the mass media practically since their inception, but it was in magazines that the first advertisement aimed at a national audience appeared. As magazines have become more and more specialized, television now captures the largest share of advertising revenue and allows advertisers to reach the most people.

Advertising occurs in more venues than the mass media, but the media receive about 60 percent of the approximately $200 billion spent annually on advertising in the United States. The remainder goes toward other advertising activities such as direct marketing, sales promotion, and package design.

Direct-to-Consumer Pharmaceutical Advertising

In advertisements directly related to health and health care, an area of significant growth during the past decade has been DTC advertising of pharmaceuticals and medical services. However, the practice is as old as advertising itself and has always been a subject of criticism.

Snake oil salesmen sold products by advertising claims to cure almost any human ailment. Exhibit 5.1 shows a 19th-century advertisement for Dr. Kilmer's Swamp Root Kidney Liver and Bladder Cure, which claimed to "relieve and cure" Bright's disease, rheumatism, diabetes, and other liver and kidney ailments. The early success of advertising claiming health benefits from the use of a product proved effective. One notable example is the success of Lydia Pinkham, who made a concoction of herbs, seeds, roots—and alcohol. She initially gave it away to her friends, but after a small promotional effort and an ad in the *Boston Herald*, the potion caught

Exhibit 5.1. Nineteenth-Century Advertisement: Dr. Kilmer's Swamp Root Kidney Liver and Bladder Cure.

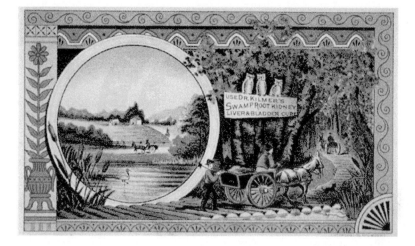

on, claiming to relieve "female complaints." That small start rolled into a nationwide advertising campaign that used newspapers as well as signs painted on barns, houses, and large rocks (DeFleur & Dennis, 2002).

Pharmaceutical companies today are well aware of the lessons of the power of advertising that early entrepreneurs such as Lydia Pinkham and her family discovered. Much of that power is through subtle rather than direct appeals to consumers. For example, Viagra advertisements never mention the penis or sexual intercourse. Instead, in one representative advertisement, a handsome middle-aged, conservatively dressed couple is seen gracefully dancing; they must be married; they are in love even after all those years together; they are a family. Viagra, the ad implies, has done all that for them.

In 1997 the U.S. Food and Drug Administration issued a guidance on mass media promotion of prescription drugs that relaxed the rules regarding the promotion of prescription drugs on television and radio. Although it still does not match the amount of money pharmaceutical companies spend on direct-to-provider marketing and free samples, the result has been a rapid increase in the amount of DTC advertisements in all the mass media.

In contrast, the European Union member nations and most other nations around the world do not allow DTC advertising of pharmaceuticals. In fact, the United States and New Zealand, as of this writing, are the only industrialized nations that allow DTC advertising of prescription drugs. However, a report by senior academic staff from all four of New Zealand's medical schools urged a ban on this advertising (Burton, 2003), and the New Zealand Ministry of Health is reportedly seeking a ban on DTC advertising by 2006.

In the United States, over half of the money spent on DTC advertising in 2000 was to promote just 20 products; the top 10 were Vioxx, Prilosec, Claritin, Paxil, Zocor, Viagra, Celebrex, Flonase, Allegra, and Meridia (Rosenthal, Berndt, Donohue, Frank, & Epstein, 2002). DTC advertising seems to have had the desired impact from the pharmaceutical company's point of view. One in five Americans reported that DTC advertising prompted them to visit or call their doctor to discuss an advertised drug, according to a PharmTrends survey by Ipsos-NPD (Gottlieb, 2002). In 2002, a marketing expert was quoted as estimating that the average American sees nine advertisements for prescription drugs on television each day (Mintzes, 2002). In 1999, the increase in sales for the 24 most advertised drugs accounted for 34 percent of the total increase in retail spending on prescription drugs (Findlay, 2001).

Analysis and reactions to DTC advertising are mixed. Overall, this approach to advertising has been viewed as:

- Making consumers aware of new drugs and the conditions they treat

- Increasing patient demands for explanations of the claims made

- Increasing consumer demand for certain drugs

- Contributing to an increase in the amount of prescription drugs dispensed

- Raising revenues for pharmaceutical companies

- Contributing to higher pharmaceutical costs for health insurers, governments, and consumers

DTC advertisements require a more health-literate audience to accurately and judiciously interpret the claims made. The demands placed on health literacy skills span the domains of health literacy put forth in this book: fundamental, cultural, civic, and scientific.

A number of questions have to be asked about DTC advertising:

- Do the advertisements lead to the appropriate treatment?

- Do the advertisements lead to the choice of more expensive drugs?

- Do the advertisements provide balanced information to aid in good decision making?

- Do the advertisements promote drug use among healthy people?

- Will the revenue generated allow pharmaceutical companies to develop new drugs to treat the diseases that harm human health the most, or will they create further incentives to overfocus on common but not life-threatening diseases such as baldness or sexual dysfunction?

- Do the advertisements market through the use of fear?

- Should the advertisements and pharmaceutical companies be allowed to "medicalize" normal human conditions and risks such as baldness?

- Should DTC advertising for clinical tests and services such as genetic testing be allowed, considering the complexity of the information, the social and cultural controversy surrounding genetics, and a lack of complete consensus about the clinical utility of some tests?

Product Placement

Another form of advertising, particularly found in films, is product placement. This is the deliberate placement of a product in a scene or image. In films, product manufacturers or businesses usually pay to have their branded product placed in the films. In television, the Federal Communications Commission requires paid placement to be disclosed during the program, so companies have found a loophole by supplying their products for free.

Areas of specific health concern related to product placement include the use of tobacco and alcohol. The practices are not new. For example, the National Coalition on TV Violence monitored 150 films in 1989 and found tobacco use in 83 percent and alcohol consumption in 93 percent of the films.

With the advent of technology such as TiVo that allows TV viewers to skip advertisements, there is a growing concern that placement will become more common. *Salon* magazine reported on an episode of *Will and Grace* on NBC in April 2001 during which viewers were solicited to "buy the shirt" off star Debra Messing's back through a ten-second spot plugging the Polo shirt. Each shirt sold at the Polo Web site would result in a $15 contribution to "programs dedicated to raising cancer awareness." According to *Salon*, the promotion resulted in a doubling of traffic on Polo's Web site; 3,000 shirts were sold, raising more than $45,000 for cancer research as well as $110,000 for Polo, which, according to *Salon*, was half owned by NBC at the time.

Those types of partnerships raise a number of ethical questions, especially when the mass media content is aimed at children. Perhaps the most famous product placement is from the 1982 movie *ET*, when the alien discovered a passion for Reese's Pieces. Today children's television programs are heavily tied to product licensing arrangements, in part an effect of the growing trend toward consolidation of media ownership into entertainment companies such as Disney or Warner Brothers.

Wrapping Up

The mass media—television, radio, newspapers, magazines, books, and the internet (discussed in the next chapter)—have and will continue to play a critically important role in linking individuals with information about their own, their family's, and their community's health. That role will only increase in the future as new technologies continue to make it easier and more affordable to deliver vast amounts of information to large numbers of people quickly. This chapter provided an overview of the traditional mass media, an area ripe with implications for health literacy, as many of the following case studies will demonstrate in further detail.

Exercises

1. Look at last week's front pages and the front of the Health section in the *New York Times*. How many articles are there about health that made it to page 1? What about those articles do you think moved them to page 1 versus the articles that were in the Health section? Are any controversies about health presented? If so, is it clear what health care decisions readers should make?

2. Select one article from the *New York Times* coverage used in exercise 1. Now look for articles about the same topic in different newspapers and magazines or on television. How do different media outlets cover the same story? Why do you think they are different or the same?

3. Write a press release about a health issue that interests you. How will you try to interest journalists in the story?

6

Health Literacy and the Internet

Mary's doctor just told her that her son Mark has "a mild case" of pneumonia and wants to keep him in the hospital overnight. Although the doctors and nurses do not seem to be terribly concerned, Mary is beside herself with fear and anxiety. While coming home to gather a few items for Mark's stay in the hospital, Mary decides to spend a few minutes on the internet to learn about pneumonia. She searched on the word *pneumonia* and after making her way past a web site for a band called "Rockin' Pneumonia," Mary finds a site that claims to focus on "Kids' Health for Parents." Quickly skimming through the pages of information about pneumonia, Mary now has more questions and fewer answers about what caused her son's pneumonia. She dashes back to the hospital, prepared to question the doctors and nurses about her son's condition.

Mary is one of the millions of adults in the United States who have used the internet to find health or medical information (Fox & Rainie, 2000). Throughout this chapter, we will return to Mary's story, a fictional one, in order to highlight some of the health literacy issues the internet presents.

Today most books on communication have a section dealing with the internet and other new media. Fifty years ago, when the first seeds of the ideas that became the internet were just beginning to sprout, the previous sentence was closer to science fiction than nonfiction. Nevertheless, many of the fundamental health literacy challenges that are true of the traditional mass media are also true for the internet. This chapter will point out the potential benefits, and limitations, of using the internet to communicate health information and the health literacy challenges that accompany this newest mass medium.

The internet, like television, radio, newspapers, and the printing press, has and will continue to have a significant role and impact on what people talk about and how they talk about it. That impact will be both positive and negative and will continue to be surrounded by debate, controversy, continuing studies, and a lack of complete understanding.

Internet Use in Health Care

During a study we recently conducted on how low-literate women make use of the internet, one participant sat down at a computer and ventured onto the internet for the very first time. She exclaimed, "Wow! You can click on just about anything you want to know." She sharply drew her breath in as the next page appeared. "Wow, oh this is so cool, if I learn," she said. "I wish I had a computer. Wow" (Zarcadoolas, Blanco, Boyer, & Pleasant, 2002).

Information is now globally delivered at amazing speeds to millions of people. E-mail exchanges, chatrooms, and listservs are bringing people together with other people and information in new and often unexpected ways. On a fundamental level, the novelty of the internet is compelling even to those who have never accessed it, and a majority of the citizens of the world have not. While physical access issues are well documented, generally under the rubric of digital divide, there is less of an understanding of how nonmainstream populations use or will use the internet after access to the internet is in place.

Who Uses the Internet

In the United States, there are roughly 2 million new internet users every month. According to the U.S. Census Bureau, more than half of U.S. households in 2003 had a computer (61.8 percent) and are using the internet (54.6 percent), with nearly one-quarter (19.9 percent) having broadband (high-speed) internet access (National Telecommunications and Information Administration, 2004). In early 2002, roughly 605 million people around the globe were accessing the internet for information ranging from telephone numbers to "free" sex, from health tips to quack cures. The vast majority of those users are located in the United States and Canada (182.67 million), Europe (190.91 million), and Asia/Pacific region countries (187.24 million) (Table 6.1).

A digital divide clearly exists both within and between nations, prompting calls for action to reduce and eliminate inequitable access. Most often describing the gap between those who are accessing and using computers and the internet and those who are not,

Table 6.1. Estimated Internet Access, 2002.

Region	Number of Internet Users (million)	Total Population	Estimated Internet Access (%)
World	605.6	More than 6 billion	10
Canada and United States	182.67	316 million	58
Europe, including Commonwealth of Independent States	190.91	727 million	26
Latin America	33.35	520 million	7
Asia/Pacific	187.24	3.7 billion	5
Africa	6.31	795 million	Less than 1

Sources: Kuruvilla et al. (2004); http://www.nua.ie/surveys/how_many_online/.

the digital divide is a well-documented phenomenon especially affecting low-income, low-literate consumers and speakers of languages other than English (National Telecommunications and Information Administration, 2004). According to a National Science Board (NSB) report (2002), while internet access is increasing for all demographic groups within the United States, access is greatest for people with the most income and education and is more common among Asian Americans and whites than blacks and Hispanics. On a positive note, the report agrees that use rates are rising fastest among black and Hispanic households.

Some believe the digital divide is bridged when computers and connectivity are installed. However, it is more often the case that the true meaning of the divide only becomes apparent when the technology arrives. Ownership and management of the infrastructure, technology, and content also contribute to the divide. These aspects of the digital divide tend to reflect existing social and economic divides (Kuruvilla et al., 2004).

Future increases in numbers of users will not simply be a matter of hardware access. The manner in which content is presented on the internet will also affect the number of users. Much of the content currently requires a high level of reading comprehension skills, generally 12th grade or higher. Individuals who are low literate or speakers of languages other than English are the most negatively affected by the current state of health and other information on internet.

What the Internet Is Used For

Mary has several questions about the source of her son's pneumonia prompted by the web site's description of the infection. The web site said pneumonia can be caused by a variety of microorganisms, including viruses, bacteria, and parasites. Mary was immediately worried that maybe she had not kept her home clean enough or that Mark may have picked up the infection at school or from friends. She wondered what she should do to prevent this in the future. The web site also told her that pneumonia caused by bacteria was different than if a virus was the cause. While she was not entirely sure about the difference, she wanted to know what caused her son's pneumonia. Mary was happy she found the web site, but the information she encountered did not leave her feeling any better informed.

A U.S. National Telecommunications and Information Agency (NTIA) study (2004) found that the main use of the internet was for e-mail, followed by searching for a product and then accessing news, weather, and sports information. Accessing information related to health was the fifth most frequently reported activity, with shopping being the fourth most reported activity (National Telecommunications and Information Administration, 2004; Figure 6.1). Women are frequently found to use the internet for health information more than men, one of the few content areas where women are more frequent users (Eysenbach, Sa, & Diepgen, 1999).

The internet seems to be put to good use as a source of health-related information, but the picture is not entirely clear. A public opinion poll in August 2001 concluded that almost 100 million American adults regularly go online for information about health care (Harris Interactive, 2001). Another survey conducted by the Pew Internet and American Life Project (2005) found that 8 in 10 internet users have looked for health information online, 82 percent of women and 75 percent of men using the internet are health seekers, and 27 percent have a high school diploma or less formal education. That same survey found that the most frequent health-seeking activity is to find information about a specific disease or medical problem, followed by information about a certain medical procedure (Table 6.2).

However, researchers looking at the words people use on search engines found that less than 1 percent of the top 300 search terms were health related (Phillipov & Phillips, 2003). In a similar study using a different data source, Eysenbach and Kohler (2004) found that 3.6 to 5.3 percent of search terms are health related.

Figure 6.1. Online Activities as a Percentage of Internet Users, Persons Age Three and Up, 2001.

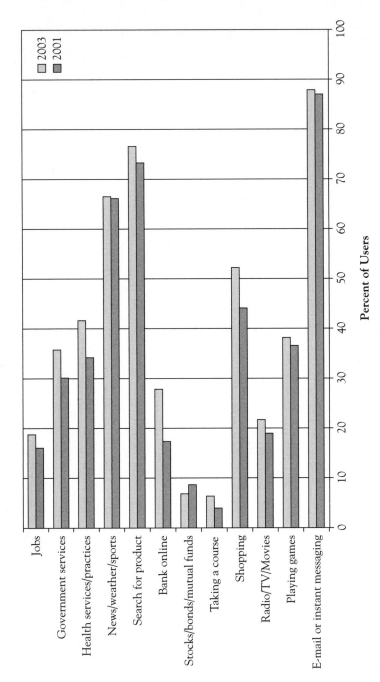

■ 2003
■ 2001

Percent of Users

Source: National Telecommunications and Information Administration (2004).

Table 6.2. Health Topics Searched Online.

Health Topic	Internet Users Who Have Searched for Information on It (%)	
	2002	2004
Specific disease or medical problem	63%	66%
Certain medical treatment or procedure	47	51
Diet, nutrition, vitamins, or nutritional supplements[a]	44	51
Exercise or fitness[a]	36	42
Prescription or over-the-counter drugs[a]	34	40
Health insurance[a]	25	31
Alternative treatments or medicines	28	30
A particular doctor or hospital[a]	21	28
Depression, anxiety, stress, or mental health issues	21	23
Experimental treatments or medicines[a]	18	23
Environmental health hazards	17	18
Immunizations or vaccinations	13	16
Sexual health information	10	11
Medicare or Medicaid	9	11
Problems with drugs or alcohol	8	8
How to quit smoking	6	7

Note: The typical health seeker has searched for five topics. About a third of health seekers have searched for seven or more topics.

[a]Statistically significant differences. The margin of error for comparing the two samples is ± 4.6 percent.

Source: Pew Internet and American Life Project (2005, p. i).

Despite that apparent contradiction, which is mainly a result of different approaches to measuring use of the internet to find information about health, it is important to remember that even 3 percent of the millions of internet searches that occur is a very large number of information requests. In addition, there is no reason to believe that the search engines used in the search word analyses reported above are reflective of all search engines or that all people use search engines when looking for information about health. Finally, most of the physicians we have talked to mention how commonplace it is for patients to come into their offices with information they have downloaded from the internet. The internet is going to continue to play a growing role in the day-to-day lives of people around the world.

Health Information on the Internet

When she first sat down at the computer, Mary was unsure if she would find anything useful about pneumonia in the short time that she had available to search. She had talked about the internet with her family and friends, and most people seemed to think there is a lot of information to access, but it was hard to tell what was good and what was bad. Plus, a lot of people Mary knew had trouble reading the web pages, sometimes because the page didn't look right and sometimes because the information didn't seem very clear.

She felt as if the web site she found contained some good information about pneumonia, but she wasn't sure how to tell, so she was eager to talk to the doctors and nurses at the hospital about what she found out.

People are turning to the internet for information about their health. When they get there, according to a study released in 1999, an estimated 100,000 sites offer health-related information (Eysenbach et al., 1999). Sheer numbers alone, however, do not tell the entire tale, as the central issue about the use of the internet for health care should be not about quantity but about quality.

Hurricane Katrina:
People Turn to the Internet for Help

Hurricane Katrina devastated the infrastructure of the city of New Orleans and much of the surrounding Gulf coast in the fall of 2005. While there was no power within those affected areas for weeks in some places, those who fled found themselves turning with increasing frequency to the internet to find family and friends and information (Digital Divide Network, 2005).

Individuals used the web to locate and inform on another at a time when official sources of information were failing to do so. The *Los Angeles Times* quoted Jeffrey Cole, director of the University of Southern California's Annenberg School for Communication's Center for the Digital Future, as saying, "I think this will be viewed as the first event that demonstrates what the web has become in terms of being transformational in people's lives" (Gaither & Gold, 2005, para. 5).

The numbers and personal anecdotes back that up. The Red Cross reported receiving over half a billion dollars in donations over the internet. Large news sites like MSNBC.com and Yahoo News all reported the busiest days in their history. Many media outlets are also increasingly accommodating citizen journalists by allowing them to post information and photos, and to comment on those posted by others. CNN reported receiving more than 30,000 accounts and 1,500 videos or photos in a matter of days.

In addition, local newspapers and television stations in New Orleans, without a local audience or working printing presses or transmitters, quickly turned to the internet as their medium of distribution. The *New Orleans Times-Picayune* published three electronic-only editions at its web site, http://www.Nola.com. According to the Southern Newspaper Association (2005), hundreds of thousands of people visited the web site and viewed more than 72 million pages. People from New Orleans and now living elsewhere, as well as those around the world concerned about the tragedy, turned to the internet.

Health information runs the gamut from a high-quality, relatively easy-to-read and easy-to-access health information provider such as Healthfinder (http://www.healthfinder.gov) to the range of attempted scams hoping to separate people from their money through claims of healthy outcomes, many of which recall the patent medicines of the 1800s. Beginning with snake-oil salesmen and continuing forward to diet fads and undocumented claims about some herbal supplements, health practices have always been subject to potentially fraudulent commercial claims. The internet simply places an old challenge into a new environment. Concern about the quality (accuracy, readability, usability, and applicability) of health information on the internet is justifiably high.

How Health Information on the Internet Is Interpreted and Used

Given concerns about the quality of health information on the internet, a useful stream of research is investigating how information on the internet is used and interpreted (Bessell et al., 2002; Zarcadoolas et al., 2002). As the medium itself is relatively new, the methods researchers have developed to study the medium are also new and remain under development. However, a broad range of preliminary investigations enables a basic understanding of how people who have access to the internet interact with the information, the sources of information, and the design elements they encounter.

For example, one meta-analysis looked at the data from 10 comparative studies evaluating the effectiveness of using the internet to deliver programs to create healthier behavior. The general conclusion of this research effort is that while we are beginning to understand the amount and type of information that users collect on the internet, we do not know much about the effects of that information (Bessell et al., 2002).

Other studies have found that internet users value personal stories as well as professional sites. This can lead to the unfortunate result that some users are not distinguishing between commercial and independent information. Internet users are urged to and often say they judge credibility by looking at the source of information, the quality of the design, and factors such as the number of external links on a site. However, when actual use is observed, users rarely check the specific pages that describe the source of information on a web site (for example, pages called "about us").

As any practicing physician can now tell you, to the chagrin of many and the delight of some, a flood of information is regularly arriving with patients as they visit their doctors. Patients are bringing questions about or seeking validation of the information they encounter on the internet on a regular basis. This is clearly one of the many changes in current health care practices affecting the nature of the doctor-patient relationship in particular; in the past, only the most proactive of patients would get access to medical information beyond that discussed by family, friends, and other lay sources of information.

Opportunities and Cautions

Every communication medium has its own distinct set of opportunities and barriers. While we have already identified inequitable access to information as an existing problem, there are several clear opportunities to this new mass medium. The internet offers health care professionals and health communication practitioners a new means to communicate with patients and others seeking information, particularly by supplying information on demand. The internet allows a patient or consumer to retrieve information without waiting for a face-to-face encounter with a provider, increasing the relevance and likelihood of retaining and acting on information by providing it just-in-time. Of course, each possible advantage to the internet comes with a caution (Table 6.3).

Potential Disadvantages and Barriers to the Internet for Conveying Health-Related Information

Eysenbach (2000, p. 1) wrote that "the principal dilemma of the internet is that its anarchic nature is desirable as it fosters open debate without censorship, but at the same time it raises quality

Table 6.3. Opportunities and Cautions of the Internet.

Opportunity	Caution
Improved access to personalized health information	Privacy concerns are very real when placing or distributing personal information on the Internet.
Access to health information, support, and services on demand.	Information without proper context and guidance can be misunderstood.
Just-in-time information	Communication using an Internet-based interface can be less effective than face-to-face interpersonal communication.
More choices for consumers	Some choices may not be good. Freedom and availability of choice require an informed decision-making process in order to result in positive outcomes.
Ability to provide information in a manner suitable to various literacy levels	A solid argument can and has been made that it makes greater sense to present all information in an easy-to-read manner. Simply because members of the audience may, for example, possess a college-level education does not mean that they will not appreciate and benefit from simple, clear, concise, and easy-to-read and easy-to-understand written and visual information. However, a goal of making information easier to access and read should not be taken as a justification to provide less information or to leave out the proper caveats and cautions that inherently accompany scientific information about health.

Opportunity	Caution
Enhanced ability to distribute materials widely and rapidly update content or functions	Rapid updating does not mean chasing the "flavor of the day." This places a special burden on Internet-based information providers to clearly indicate the efficacy of their claims and provide links to competing, and contradicting, information when it is present.
An opportunity to democratize knowledge, making information widely available	Just because health information is available to all does not mean that all health information is equal. Equity can come in the form of equal access to information, but inequity can come from equal access to unequal information.

problems that could inhibit its potential." While that dilemma is very real, we feel the barriers and disadvantages of the internet as a source of health information are surmountable through appropriate planning, appropriation of resources, and careful goal setting by health communicators. This will require an application of the principles of health literacy outlined in this book along with technically competent web design skills. In this section, we discuss some of the major concerns about the internet, especially those grounded in concerns about health literacy, and how they can be addressed.

Complex Language

There is only a small but growing body of theoretical or empirical work examining the complexity of internet-based information (Haas & Grams, 2000; Graber, Roller, & Kaeble, 1999). However, the literacy level and formats in which topics are presented on the internet are relatively high as compared to the literacy level of the U.S. and global population. Almost 50 percent of the U.S. population reads at or below the eighth-grade level (Kirsch et al., 1993), while most health information is written at the 10th-grade level and higher (Zarcadoolas et al., 2005). The problems created by complex language can partially be addressed through the use of plain language techniques and simple sentence structures (see Chapter 4), but if so-called plain language is presented through a complex and difficult-to-navigate web site, the information is still difficult to find and use.

Difficulty Navigating

On the internet, important literacy skills include the abilities to read as well as navigate the design of web sites. Hurdles to successful navigation are many, and we identify specific strategies to make web sites more accessible in Chapter 13. In addition, visual and physical disabilities can hinder access to information available through the range of information and communication technologies. In the United States, federal agencies are required to ensure accessibility to be in compliance with the standards established in Section 508 of the Rehabilitation Act (see http://www.usability.gov and http://www.section508.gov). Many of those standards are also incorporated in the slightly more rigorous accessibility standards established by the World Wide Web Consortium (available at http://www.w3.org/WAI). Several web sites offer to check the accessibility of web sites somewhat automatically, often tied to a labeling scheme to indicate that the site is fully accessible. Examples that are currently free to use (versus those that require registration or a fee) include "Cynthia says" at http://www.contentquality.com/, HI Software (includes privacy check) at http://www.hisoftware.com/accmonitorsitetest/, and the WEBSAT analyzer tool at http://zing.ncsl.nist.gov/WebTools/WebSAT/overview.html.

Dominance of English

The delivery of words, pictures, and sounds over the internet is mainly conducted using a computer language, hypertext markup language, but the majority of information that users see remains in English. This limits the information that non-English speakers may access and use, and it limits the participation and input from a majority of the world's population. In short, information on the internet is written not only at too high of a level but also in too few languages. Establishing an internet site only in English is akin to opening a chain of department stores around the world but hiring only English-speaking employees. However, efficiency and economics, put in perspective of the trend toward English as the dominant language of science and business, can argue in favor of a single language. As with many other issues, the decision rests on values.

Complex Scientific Information

Complexity in science lies not only in the nature of the questions science attempts to answer, but also in how the scientific information is presented (see the case studies on anthrax and genomics in Chapters 8 and 9, respectively.) On a broad scale, the American public does not have a thorough understanding of how science works or know some of the fundamental knowledge produced by the scientific method. For example, the U.S. National Science Board's *Science and Engineering Indicators* report (2004) contains, in part, the results of a telephone survey of a sample of the American public. Two open-ended questions, one about probability and another about the design of a medical experiment, are included in the annual survey. In the several years that each question has been asked, no more than 39 percent of the participants correctly explained an experiment, and no more than 57 percent of participants correctly answered the question on probability. In addition, roughly half of the participants in a random sample telephone survey participants incorrectly responded to the statement, "The earliest humans lived at the same time as the dinosaurs." (The correct answer is false.)

Questionable Accuracy and Timeliness of Information

Problems with health information on the internet can develop through source bias, source distortion, and self-serving information, among others. There are currently no universally effective or applied means to patrol the internet for misinformation, inaccuracies, or out-dated information. Arguments for content regulation are countered by the threat of regulation to the valued ability of the internet to offer easy entry for all points of view into the public discussion. Many of the positions in the debates over regulating internet content are based on values, so discussion is likely to endure without resolution. However, from a health literacy perspective, it is clear that the potential negative impact of misleading and inaccurate information poses a significant problem for less literate users.

Conflicting Information

Science is often a process of resolving conflicting evidence and claims. Health and medical information is certainly no exception. From television news to newspapers and internet-based coverage of health, the latest reported research findings often contradict earlier research. For instance, one study found conflicting health informa-tion on over half of the internet sites reviewed (Berland et al., 2001). Distinguishing worthy from unworthy claims is difficult enough for high-literate individuals, and that challenge is com-pounded for those with lower literacy skills and little or no under-standing of the scientific process.

Inappropriate Framing and Content

Anyone can go virtually anywhere on the internet with few restric-tions. Efforts should be made to notify those visiting web sites about whom the site is intended for and what type and level of health in-formation they will encounter. This is rarely accomplished, but is beginning to be found on some government web sites such as Med-lineplus (http://www.nlm.nih.gov/medlineplus/), which is labeling some information as easy to read, or targeted to senior citizens, or in Spanish. Providing descriptions in advance of delivering infor-mation is one means of assisting those with low health literacy in their search for useful information. A potential triple difficulty of poor health communication practices can occur on the internet when complex language requiring a high literacy level is present, there is not a mirror site in alternative languages, and the framing or content is inappropriate to the audience.

Local Unavailability of Services

Imagine that a person recently diagnosed with a serious illness goes to the internet for information and treatment options. After spending hours searching, she discovers a health care facility that offers treatment services and health products that promise effective relief. However, just as she experiences the exhilaration at finding exactly what she was looking for, she discovers that the facility is located far away or that she is not allowed to purchase the health products in her country.

Equally unproductive situations involve children being exposed to medical information their parents find inappropriate, or a health care facility placing information on the internet that offends the ethics or religious codes of individuals seeking health care. While the nature of the internet makes addressing these problems difficult, it is not impossible. To not make the attempt to address potential negative issues associated with placing health care information on the internet is to unwittingly create disincentives for individuals to seek health care and information when they need it.

Privacy Issues

One of the most discussed issues about the internet is the potential for invasion of generally private domains of behavior and information use. The technology easily lends itself to tracking movement within and between sites on the internet. Furthermore, in the effort to better understand behavior and make more sales on the internet, there is an explosion of requests for personal information. At least one study has found that while individuals are aware of privacy concerns, a majority of internet users have provided sites with personal information (Eysenbach et al., 1999). This technologically based potential for invasion of privacy is often accompanied by privacy statements or disclaimers. However, those statements are usually written in language too complex for most people to understand.

Consider this sample privacy statement:

> Only statistical information about our visitors as a group (usage habits, demographics) may be shared with any partner of drkoop.com. Personally identifiable information will not be shared at any time without the visitor's permission. drkoop.com employs strict security measures to safeguard online transactions; personal information is stored in a secured database and always sent via an encrypted internet channel [http://www.drkoop.com/contents/93/privacy.html].

This example contains complicated notions many readers will not understand—for example, who is a partner, what demographics are referred to, what a secured database is, and what an encrypted internet channel is. But some sites, such as Doctor.com (http://www.doctor.com), do not appear to have privacy statements at all, or if they do, they are so hidden the average user will never find them.

Lack of Accountability for Advertising Claims

There is no approval process required before an individual or organization establishes a site on the internet. A relatively small initial investment in software, hardware, and storage is all that is required. As a result, commercial sites claiming health outcomes for everything from shark cartilage to urine therapy are frequent and common. Many of these claims are fraudulent or misleading; some are downright dangerous. In fact, one study found that between 50 and 90 percent of health-related information found through internet search engines was judged to contain incorrect clinical information by a panel of 34 physicians (Berland et al., 2001).

Ethical Issues

Mass media that generally rely on point sources for distribution, such as television, newspapers, and magazines, are easier to regulate than a diffuse network structure that makes up the internet. It seems unlikely that a broad-based regulatory agency for content on the internet will be developed or found acceptable. The design of such an attempt is difficult to conceive, and the notion goes against the spirit of the internet. Areas of public health and safety, however, are likely to draw the most critical attention and demands for regulation.

One means of improving the accuracy, quality, and usability of health information on the internet is through adherence to codes of conduct or ethical guidelines. Numerous ethical guidelines have been proposed, many of them already in use. While none offers a complete solution to the dilemmas posed by the internet, to varying degrees each has its advantages and disadvantages. Perhaps the greatest weakness is in the lack of enforceability or penalties for noncompliance. Furthermore, the impact on internet users of logos indicating some form of approval of the content is not well documented. Nonetheless, the general idea seems to offer a means of ensuring some level of accuracy, completeness, and privacy that is otherwise lacking. (For a thorough analysis, see the survey of guidelines for internet content in Risk & Dzenowagis, 2001, http://www.jmir.org/2001/4/e28/.)

Another potential solution to the problem of low or no regulatory power is to establish a health information–specific domain on the internet, identified by the ending domain name of ".health." This proposal, which largely originated from the World Health Organization's Health InterNetwork project, suggests that the nonprofit organization created to establish and manage internet domains, the Internet Corporation for Assigned Names and Numbers, establish a top-level internet domain (such as .com or .biz) for trustworthy health information. The proposal would address the lack of regulatory power through an ability to suspend or withdraw the domain name in a case of noncompliance. There are ongoing discussions about who should be in control of internet domain names, and until that is resolved, the establishment of a domain such as .health may have to wait.

Wrapping Up

A communication effort without full awareness of exactly whom the message is intended for is most likely an ineffective communication effort. Just as all individuals have their particular contexts, each audience also has distinct media use patterns and capabilities. The internet, like all other communication media, has appropriate uses. An indiscriminate use of the varied information and communication technologies related to the internet will prove neither efficient nor equitable. While the internet may appear an attractive bandwagon at the moment, it is a mistake to characterize it as a one-size-fits-all solution. In fact, the technology does promise to greatly enhance the relationship of individuals with the health care system and individual health care providers, but all bandwagons should be treated with caution.

Exercises

1. Divide into groups, and select a health topic. Each individual in each group should go to the internet and find information on that topic. Later, compare strategies for searching and the results. Did everyone use the same strategy? Do the results agree?

2. Go to the web site of your local hospital, if it has one. How easy is it to find answers to the following questions:

Where is the hospital located?

How can I get there? What if I don't have a car?

How do I make an appointment to get a flu shot?

Can I get my children's vaccinations there?

Must I have insurance to see a doctor?

I speak only Spanish. Is there any information on the web site I can understand?

3. Look on the internet for information about any prescription drug recently advertised on television. What sort of information do you find? Is it easy to read? Can you purchase the medication over the internet? Discuss how people are to decide if they need the medication, how to obtain the medication, and what risks and side effects are associated with the medication.

Internet Jargon Unwrapped

Chat—live communication by computer between two or more users.

Cookie—A message given to a web browser (such as Netscape Navigator or Internet Explorer) by the web site (specifically the web server). These are most frequently used to identify users and customize web pages for visitors.

Domain—an area of jurisdiction on the internet, with domain names organized by type of organization sponsoring the web site. Current domain names include .com,

Internet Jargon Unwrapped, *continued*

commercial entities and businesses; .edu, educational institutions; .gov, U.S. government; .net, internet organizations; and .org, nonprofit organizations and other groups.

E-mail—Short for electronic mail, this is the transmission of messages between computers over a network such as the internet.

HTML (hypertext markup language)—A language used to create web pages. Commands, or words, in the language tell a web browser what to display.

Hyperlink—A function of HTML that allows documents or web pages to be linked together. Typically, clicking on the hyperlink connects users to the new content.

ICT—Information and communication technologies. Can refer to new technology such as the internet or wireless devices, as well as to old technology such as radio and the telephone.

Internet—A network of computer networks. A network is two or more computers connected together. The internet facilitates data transmission providing a variety of media services: text, video, audio, and graphics.

IP address—A specific address for a specific computer on a specific network.

PDF (portable document format)—Developed by Adobe Systems, PDF allows users to open a document in a range of hardware and software and have it still look the same.

Surfing—The act of following links on the World Wide Web to see what can be found.

Web browser—A software package that can read and display the page as indicated by HTML.

Web server—A computer that serves a web page to browsers when requested. Most any computer can be made a server by loading the correct software and attaching the computer to the internet.

World Wide Web (WWW)—A system of internet servers that supports delivery of hypertext and multimedia.

7

Baby Basics

A Prenatal Program Focusing on Developing Health Literacy

Baby Basics is a prenatal health literacy program that addresses health disparities and poor birth outcomes by helping health care providers and educators fully engage and empower low-income pregnant women. At the launch of a citywide Baby Basics initiative in Houston, Texas, in 2004, U.S. Surgeon General Vice Admiral Richard Carmona said:

> Often there was a wall between us and the people we were trying to serve. It was a wall of confusion and mis-understanding brought on by low functional literacy skills. And, unfortunately, it was sometimes shored up by our inability to recognize that our patients didn't under-stand the health information that we were trying to communicate. We must close the gap between what health care professionals know and what the rest of America understands about how to have a healthy preg-nancy and a healthy baby. Not every American is a sci-entist or a health care professional, and we can't expect

This chapter was prepared with the assistance of Shusmita Dhar and Lisa Bernstein. The pilot and evaluation activities described in this chapter were partially funded by a grant from the Altman Foundation of New York City.

everyone to understand what it takes doctors, nurses, pharmacists, and other health care professionals years of training to learn. That's why the Baby Basics Program is so important.

This case highlights the importance of developing health education materials that are matched with respect to language and culture and using that material to its full potential. It also demonstrates that collaborating and continuously working with target audiences and communities is vital in producing effective health promotion strategies and the specific communications for patients as well as providers.

Healthy Beginnings: Infant and Maternal Health

For many underserved women, prenatal care is the entry point into the health care system. For some first-time expectant women, the initial prenatal appointment is the first time she will visit an obstetrician/gynecologist. It is critical to help a pregnant woman access and understand the need for early and consistent care (in 2001 in the United States, one out of nine births was to women receiving late or no prenatal care). Helping a woman to make pregnancy lifestyle changes and to engage fully in her prenatal care is crucial. It will have an impact on birth outcomes and influence her abilities to manage her own and her newborn's health care.

The preventable death of an infant is one of the great tragedies of life. The overall U.S. infant mortality rate decreased to 6.8 percent in 2001 largely due to factors including improved fetal screening, mothers adopting protective behaviors such as not smoking, placing children on their backs to sleep, and increases in early enrollment for prenatal care. However, the U.S. infant mortality rate is higher than that of 27 other nations, and those in underserved communities are at greater risk. For example, black infants are more than twice as likely to die as white infants: 14.1 deaths per 1,000 live births each year versus the national average of 6.9 in 2000 (National Center for Health Statistics, 2001).

In 2001, about one in nine infants (11.3 percent of live births) was born to a woman receiving inadequate prenatal care in the United States. In a health system that is characterized by advancing technology and resources, experts point the finger at both a breakdown of prenatal service delivery and problematic health literacy on the part of pregnant mothers (National Center for Health Statistics, 2001).

Education level and literacy level correlate with prenatal health (Clenland & Van Ginniken, 1988). As a woman's literacy increases, infant mortality decreases, with lower education levels correlating to later prenatal care (PRAMS Working Group, 1997; Chang et al., 2003).

Prenatal education has been available and promoted for more than a century in the United States. While eligibility for prenatal care varies greatly nationwide, federal programs such as Healthy Start encourage prenatal health education and some form of home health care visits in communities with high infant mortality rates. Introducing the importance of good prenatal care, proper diet, and health practices during pregnancy and explaining the risks of using alcohol, tobacco, and street drugs are central in prenatal education. Most prenatal education efforts, however, do not adequately address the health literacy or the fundamental literacy levels of many pregnant women, especially low-income and ethnic minority women.

The book *What to Expect When You're Expecting* (Eisenberg, Murkoff, & Hathaway, 2002) is by far the most popular mainstream book for pregnant women, with over 26 million copies sold. The book is read by over 1 million women each year and is available in over 30 countries. It is written at an 11th- to 13th-grade level and therefore is suitable for a woman with a high-level ability to read (fundamental literacy) as well as competence in other domains of health literacy. (See Chapter 3 for a discussion of these domains.) The following passage comes from a section of the book titled, "The Father's Age":

> "I'm only 31, but my husband is over 50. Does advanced paternal age pose risks to a baby?" Throughout most of history, it was believed that a father's responsibility in the reproductive process was limited to fertilization. Only during the 20th century (too late to help those queens who lost their heads for failing to produce a male heir) was it discovered that a father's sperm held the deciding genetic vote in determining his child's gender. And only in the last few years have researchers postulated that an older father's sperm might contribute to birth defects such as Down syndrome. Like the older mother's ova, the older father's primary oocytes (undeveloped sperm) have had longer exposure to environmental hazards and might conceivably contain altered or damaged genes or chromosomes. And from the studies that have been done, there is some evidence that in about 25 or 30% of Down syndrome cases, the faulty chromosome can be traced to the father [p. 33].

The reader of this material must:

- Understand difficult vocabulary

- Read complex language and sentence structure

- Identify topics of interest

- Navigate a complicated text to find answers

- Easily adapt to switches between a formal and colloquial tone

- Appreciate the sophisticated style that has references to history and metaphorical descriptions

- Have an understanding of basic body anatomy

Fundamental Literacy

Fundamental literacy refers to the ability to read, write, speak, and work with numbers. It is a keystone of health literacy.

Written and spoken health information is full of complex language (both vocabulary and syntax).

- Health information and materials are often not tailored to end user skills and abilities in reading, writing, speaking, and numeracy.

What to Expect When You're Expecting authors Heidi Murkoff, Arlene Eisenberg, and Sandee Hathaway received continuous requests for book donations from clinics across the country that provide prenatal care and education to the Medicaid population. Lisa Bernstein, an executive at Workman Publishing with a background in commercial book marketing and materials development, as well as a volunteer literacy tutor for recovering drug addicts, identified the need for a different health promotion vehicle—one that specifically addresses fundamental literacy skills as well as the economic, cultural, and social concerns of underserved families. Eisenberg, Murkoff, and Bernstein formed the What to Expect Foundation hoping to identify or create a book similar in scope and tone to *What to Expect When You're Expecting* and was appropriate for women with low literacy levels. They created *Baby Basics: Your Month by Month Guide to a Healthy Pregnancy* (the Spanish version is titled *Hola Bebé*). Teaching providers, educators, and patients how best to use this book led to the creation of the Baby Basics Prenatal Health Literacy Program.

Providing the materials and the support needed to read and act on written health information improves care and saves health care dollars. A UCLA/Johnson & Johnson Healthcare Institute study found that when Head Start parents were provided with a comprehensive early childhood health education book and health literacy classes to help them use the book to assess appropriate care for a sick child, emergency room visits went down and annual health care costs were reduced by at least $198 per family per year ("UCLA Study," 2004).

The fundamental goals of the Baby Basics Program are to:

- Promote healthier pregnancies and safer deliveries

- Foster effective communication and partnership between providers and their patients within the prenatal health care community

- Empower pregnant women to engage and act on health information, thus learning to care for themselves and their babies

The Baby Basics Book and Program

The Baby Basics Program was developed in four phases:

Phase 1—Identify the needs of the target audience of low-income, low-literate, and underserved pregnant women by working collaboratively with them to choose content and then design appropriate materials.

Phase 2—Field-test the material with providers and pregnant mothers in the target audience.

Phase 3—Develop best practice guidelines for using *Baby Basics* based on empirical testing.

Phase 4—Create a replicable Baby Basics Prenatal Health Literacy Program model and evaluate outcomes.

Phase 1: Collaboratively Identifying the Need

In 1998, the foundation conducted an extensive audit of existing prenatal materials created for low-income women. They discovered that while high-risk women and teens may be enrolled in many programs (for example, Women, Infants, and Children [WIC], home visitation programs, and childbirth classes), these women were unlikely to receive comprehensive, coordinated health information in a manner they could understand. Many receive pamphlets and uncoordinated advice from a number of sources varying in content and language.

Existing programs mostly relied on information sheets and handouts that were poorly written and designed and thus too complicated to read and use. There was a tremendous duplication of resources and energy by individual programs from around the country and across the street, all seeking grants to develop materials that ultimately were written and designed on a limited budget and were quickly outdated. To a low-literate reader, these materials sent out all the wrong signals. Some responses to typical pamphlets given out to pregnant women in the Bronx, New York, were: "I never read these things they give us—I end up losing them or tossing them." "This looks like something they would give me at school. Just 'cause I'm having a baby doesn't mean I've gotta do homework." "Boring. Boring. Boring. That's what that is."

The foundation spent over a year creating the *Baby Basics* book and an additional six months creating a linguistically and culturally appropriate Spanish version. The format was developed after extensive focus groups with prenatal community health outreach workers and group discussions with pregnant women in the target population. This formative research identified the appropriate literacy level as well as important content, such as an explanation of Medicaid benefits, the effects of homelessness on pregnancy, and the legal rights of a mother who tests positive for drug use at delivery.

When this information had been collected from the target audience and health workers, experts in the fields of literacy, multicultural health, Medicaid benefits, and prenatal care reviewed and fine-tuned *Baby Basics*.

Baby Basics is a month-by-month pregnancy guide that is brightly colored, spiral bound, and 288 pages long (Exhibit 7.1). The book is filled with information, stories, checklists, and pictures. Side tabs provide easy navigation. There is a chapter for each of the nine months of pregnancy, as well as a chapter on postpartum care. The remaining chapters focus on nutrition, referrals, and special issues such as homelessness, miscarriage, pregnancy in prison, and

Exhibit 7.1. Cover of *Baby Basics*.

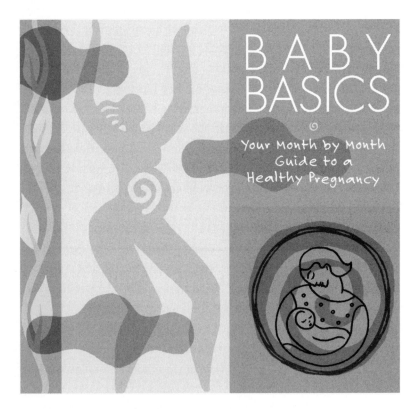

drug addiction. Each chapter has a section called "The Basics," written at a third-grade level. With fundamental literacy principles in mind, health content is color-coded and repeated to enhance comprehension and retention.

Each chapter has these sections:

"A Look At Your Baby": A month-by-month drawing and description of the fetus

"Your Changing Body": Answers the question, "Are the things I'm feeling this month normal?"

"Make a Healthy Baby": The basic medical advice women need to have each month

"Your Monthly Visit to Your Doctor or Midwife": What to expect at a checkup, questions to ask, and space to write notes (a task appropriate for those who have enough fundamental literacy skill or are writing with the help of an intermediary)

More advanced pages like the White Pages and "Take Care of Yourself" are written at approximately sixth-grade level and contain more in-depth information that builds on the "Basics" sections. For example, a "Basics" section notes that headaches are a perfectly normal symptom of pregnancy. In "Take Care of Yourself" are tips for reducing headache pain and frequency.

In addition, each chapter includes features with detailed individual experiences that help bring health information alive. "You May Have Heard" is a collection of sometimes amusing pregnancy myths, wives' tales, and cultural stories. Myths are respectfully debunked. In "Our Stories," six people share monthly pregnancy stories complete with friendly, personal tips. The wide range of their feelings and experiences ensures that some of the stories will reflect and touch the lives of many different cultures and lifestyles. For example, the following individuals contribute to the book:

- Valerie, a single mom who is unsure if congratulations are in order for her pregnancy

- Maria, a teen with a supportive boyfriend

- Amanda, an older married mom who, after a miscarriage, is joyous and nervous about this pregnancy

- Warren, an ambivalent father-to-be

- Aida, a grandmother whose young granddaughter is pregnant

- Beth, a supportive friend who worries about her friend's unhealthy lifestyle

These stories capture real-world scenarios reflective of the life situations of the target readers. As we have discussed earlier in this book, relevancy and context are key factors in communication and health literacy principles. The information must be relevant and placed in a meaningful context for readers.

The "On My Mind" section offers questions that help women become more aware of the growing baby and begin thinking of themselves as mothers. The questions are great conversation starters and promote literacy by encouraging the woman to keep a personal record of pregnancy in written and spoken language, not privileging one form of language over another.

"Tips for Dads" are spread throughout the book (and are also intended for a birth friend).

The overall tone of the book is reflective of familiar and used spoken language structures aimed at building trust (see Exhibit 7.2). For example, in month seven, friendly phrasing is ubiquitous. Under "Your Changing Body" are these comments:

"Your mind—Worries about what labor will be like"

"Forgetful; Bored with the whole thing? So excited you can't stand it."

"Your 7th Month Visit to Your Doctor or Midwife—They'll check . . . By now you know the drill. They will check . . ."

Another tonal strategy that makes the text friendly and trustworthy is the use of numerous quotations that capitalize on the power and immediacy of spoken language. For example, "Juan says my breasts are too small to breastfeed."

Phase 2: Field Testing with Providers and Pregnant Mothers

In 2002, 100,000 copies of *Baby Basics* were distributed free to programs across the United States. The only commitment necessary was that the programs agreed to return a completed evaluation form. In New York, Los Angeles County, Minneapolis, and Washington, D.C., the foundation partnered with the city health departments and invited every health care provider in each of those cities that served low-income, Medicaid-eligible pregnant women to apply for enough books for their mothers for one year. (Certain prenatal health education programs in other parts of the country, such as Early Head Start Programs, Pueblo prenatal clinics serving the Native American population, Healthy Start, and Even Start Family Literacy Programs, were also invited to apply for books.)

Exhibit 7.2. Sample Page from *Baby Basics*.

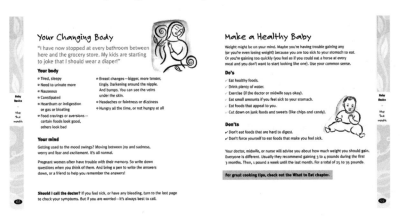

Two hundred practitioners who used *Baby Basics* were surveyed, and 20 focus groups were conducted with pregnant mothers who received *Baby Basics* from their health care provider or educator and had received it at least three months prior to meeting. The focus groups with pregnant women who had used *Baby Basics* revealed compelling insights:

- Mothers developed a relationship with *Baby Basics* because it was "beautiful" and "real." Mothers felt it was more than a handout from their nurse or doctor. It felt like a "gift." It made mothers feel special. In fact, when asked who this book was written for, 100 percent of the mothers responded that it was written "for me." When asked who they would give the book to, many mothers offered to tell their friends about it, but since some had written in the book and others felt very possessive of this gift, most said they "might lend it to someone, but I want it back, because it's mine."
- Mothers wanted to read *Baby Basics* because it had the information they wanted. One Brazilian mother proudly announced, "This is the first book I read in English from front to back. Not only was it simple, but it was exactly the information I most wanted to know. I told every one of my girlfriends to go to the clinic that had the book."
- Art matters. A 16-year-old bubbled, "It looked like a kid's book to me. Not at all scary. Something I wanted to pick up because there were bright colors and lots of pictures."
- Women finding themselves in the pages felt reassured and important. The stories in the book resonated with mothers of all ages. All of the women surveyed who had read the book had read all of the stories. A homeless mother suggested adding a story about homelessness and pregnancy: "Just knowing that other moms are in the same place as me would make me feel less alone." A mother who had recently miscarried suggested including a first-person narrative in that section too. (Both these and other suggestions were incorporated into the second edition of the book, published in 2003.)

- Some mothers needed to be coaxed or reminded to open the book, but when they did, they were happy to find the answers they wanted and surprised that a book could give them answers. A young mother said she had so many questions, "and I would ask my mom and my girlfriends and everyone told me to stop asking so many questions. Or they would all tell me something different. And the book was sitting right there near my bed, and I picked it up one night and the answers to every single one of those questions was right there. So I read the whole thing through. Twice."

Of the 200 clinicians (nurses, nurse practitioners, and health educators) surveyed who had used *Baby Basics*, 90 percent believed women in the target audience would read the book. They thought the format was appealing, and almost half surveyed believed that male partners would also read the book.

Focus groups were held with providers and health educators who received *Baby Basics* for expectant mothers. Groups of midwives, physicians, nurses, health educators, and home visitors were brought together. Focus groups found the following:

- There needed to be more of a process developed for the book's distribution and use. One clinic put the books out in the lobby, where they were quickly taken. "Our mothers love the books; they're all gone. Can we have more?"

- A group of midwives, physicians, health educators, and adult literacy teachers provided useful, insightful, and replicable ways to use the *Baby Basics* book.

- Many health care providers and educators had never considered their patients' literacy skills when providing care and had never learned how to educate patients who could not read or who read at low levels.

Phase 3: Developing Best Practice Guidelines for Using *Baby Basics*

A book alone cannot solve the health and social challenges low-income pregnant mothers face. But by watching health care professionals use *Baby Basics*, the foundation saw that the book played a role in transforming and strengthening provider-patient communications. Across the country, midwives, doctors, nurses, and educators had independently created health literacy strategies for using *Baby Basics/Hola Bebé* that changed their practice and their patients' understanding and compliance.

A series of program-building steps at health centers and cities across the country encouraged the What to Expect Foundation to develop the Baby Basics Program.

The Baby Basics Program was developed during the foundation's 2001 implementation and study of the *Baby Basics* book at the University of Medicine and Dentistry of New Jersey (UMDNJ) in Newark, New Jersey. UMDNJ houses the largest prenatal clinic in Newark, in which 79 percent of annual births (3,400 out of 4,334 deliveries) are to women living at or below poverty level (Lakota Cruse, New Jersey Maternal and Child Health Bureau statistician, private communication to the authors). High illiteracy, coupled with a high infant mortality rate of 13.2 percent, encouraged the foundation to work with Dr. Theodore Barrett Jr., assistant professor in the Department of Obstetrics, Gynecology, and Women's Health, associate chief of Ob/Gyn, and medical director at University Ob/Gyn Associates at the UMDNJ, and Jennifer Winter, the clinic's nurse manager.

At UMDNJ, every new pregnant woman attends her first prenatal appointment on a Wednesday. That session is an introduction to a "pregnancy party" that uses *Baby Basics* as an introductory tool. All mothers receive a copy in English or Spanish. They are introduced to the entire staff, and the program heads talk about their program, explain where they are located, and give the women the page numbers in *Baby Basics* that discuss the services they provide.

Mothers are told that the doctors and nurses will refer to *Baby Basics* throughout their prenatal care and that they should refer to the book for answers to their questions.

When providers and health educators who teach topics such as nutrition, breastfeeding, or labor and delivery teach at University Hospital, they do so with a copy of *Baby Basics* open on their lap or desk. Women who cannot read can look at the pictures and focus on the topics with the educator. The staff tries to use the language in *Baby Basics* in discussion. They find that "it's easier for us to all say it the same way. We know the mom hears it from all of us, and she'll start to understand we're all talking about the same thing. A c-section, a caesarean section—same thing to us, but not to a mom who has never had one and never heard the word before." Winters is enthusiastic about the program and has found that it makes her job easier: "I have it all written right in front of me. Pointing at pictures, working our way down lists, this makes sense."

At every subsequent visit, moms are told where they can find information in *Baby Basics*, reinforcing health as well as fundamental literacy skills—for example:

- Print versus spoken language: Print records information they can use as a reference, and they do not have to rely exclusively on spoken language.

- Reference: They can refer back to a written text, *Baby Basics*, for information they have heard in spoken language.

- Navigation: They can use an index to find information.

- Strategic control of vocabulary and sentence structure.

Phase 4: *Baby Basics* Toolbox for Change

In 2005, the foundation launched a program in Jamaica Queens, New York, designed to study and evaluate the Baby Basics Program and explore strategies to create a patient-centered education program that would fully integrate *Baby Basics* and health literacy strategies into prenatal care. A grant from the Altman Foundation helped the What to Expect Foundation partner with the New York City Literacy Assistance Center, Medical Health Research Associates, and the Primary Care Development Corporation to create new tools expanding the *Baby Basics* book's impact.

Baby Basics Planner

A diary that serves as pocket companion to the *Baby Basics* book has preprinted pages for a woman to track her prenatal appointments, provides a list of monthly questions, and provides space to write questions for the doctor (Exhibit 7.3). There is a space for any provider to write down *Baby Basics* page numbers to review, as well as other information moms need to remember. There is also a blank generic health form women can fill out and carry with them to other appointments.

Exhibit 7.3. Sample Page from Baby Basics Patient Planner.

2nd Month Appointment | 8-12 Weeks

DATE:

Here are some questions you may want to ask this visit. Check off those you want answered:

☐ I'm so sick. I can hardly eat. Is there something I can do?
☐ Am I gaining the right amount of weight?
☐ Is there any activity I should not do?
☐ Can you explain what the tests you are doing today are for?
☐ If I can't eat, does it hurt my baby?
☐ I'm so tired. Is this how everyone feels?

My Questions:

Look it up in *Baby Basics*. Here are pages to review at home:

TOPIC   PAGE NUMBER

Things to Remember . . .

3rd Month Appointment | 12-16 Weeks

DATE:

Here are some questions you may want to ask this visit. Check off those you want answered:

☐ What exercises are best for me to do now?
☐ The veins on my legs are getting bigger – what does that mean?
☐ Is it okay for me to keep working?
☐ I sit (or stand) all day at work. How can I help my aching back?
☐ I look bigger than my other pregnancy. Is it ok?
☐ When will the baby move?

My Questions:

Look it up in *Baby Basics*. Here are pages to review at home:

TOPIC   PAGE NUMBER

Things to Remember . . .

• 14 weeks starts your second trimester.

Baby Basics Prompt Cards

A laminated set of cards—one for each month of pregnancy, plus a postpartum card, index, and list of common complaints card—stays in each exam and education room to help providers educate patients at each visit. One side of the cards has a monthly picture of the developing fetus; the other side identifies what pages in *Baby Basics* the provider can refer patients to review later.

Baby Basics Moms Club Curriculum

This prenatal health literacy curriculum gives educators activities that reinforce prenatal education and teach fundamental literacy and health literacy skills (Exhibit 7.4). The curriculum can be used to foster supportive groups or can be used one-on-one and integrated into other case management and home visitation curricula. Skills include:

- Vocabulary mothers need to know at delivery

- How to use an index to find health information in *Baby Basics*

Exhibit 7.4. Sample from Baby Basics Moms Club Curriculum.

⑫ When to Call Your Healthcare Provider

Prenatal Goal
Make sound decisions about when to call your healthcare provider

Health Literacy Goal
Identify symptoms of labor which require a call to a healthcare provider

Materials
Baby Basics Planner (optional)

Vocabulary

emergency	rectum
vagina	bladder
swelling	bleeding
abdomen	fever
nausea	aerola
vomiting	

The Warm-Up
Ask moms who have already had a baby: When during the last pregnancy did you call the doctor? What happened? Was it helpful? Would you do the same thing, in the same situation, if it happened again?

Activity
- Read **page 292** of *Baby Basics* (*Hola Bebé*:page 286) with moms, as skills allow. As you read, list vocabulary words on the board. Read each aloud, define, read it again having moms repeat after you.

- Begin the discussion with the first story on the back of this card.

- Working in pairs, have moms discuss what they would do if they were Susie and why.

- Have moms report back.   ⟳

Exhibit 7.4. Sample from Baby Basics Moms Club Curriculum, *continued.*

12	When to Call Your Healthcare Provider
• Guide moms as necessary to refer to **page 292** to see if dark circles around breasts is a sign to call the doctor. After seeing it is not, look up breasts in the index of *Baby Basics*, then turn to **page 55** (*Hola Bebé*:page 53) and read about the dark ring around the nipple called the aerola. Discuss how moms have found what they need to know and there is no need to call a healthcare provider. • Explain there are three steps moms can take to help them decide when to call their healthcare provider, no matter what their question. Review the steps: ❶ Check **page 292**. If a symptom is there, call. If a symptom isn't there ... ❷ Look it up in the index of *Baby Basics*. Turn to the page listed. If the information you need is there, that's it. ❸ If you can't find it or need or want more information, write your question in the Baby Basics Planner or on paper that can be brought in for the next appointment.	• Have moms work in small groups and practice these steps using the stories in the **Discussion Starters** listed below or some of your favorites from the hundreds in your personal collection. As moms report back, list, define and read aloud key vocabulary words. **Discussion Starters** • As Susie was drying off after her shower, she noticed dark circles around her nipples. It was 11:00 at night. • Susie has a very bad headache that won't go away. Her head has been pounding for 3 hours. • Susie feels sick to her stomach. • Susie's hands and face are getting very puffy. What should Susie do? Go to the ER? Look it up in Baby Basics? Call her doctor? **Role Play** Have one mom be the busy nurse and have another be Susie. Help moms ask questions and respectfully demand answers.

- How to create questions to ask providers and role-playing activities to help mothers ask questions

- Ways to teach the health information necessary for most state-mandated Medicaid prenatal guidelines using adult literacy/ESOL (English for speakers of other languages) strategies for skill development

The Jamaica partnership also created a replicable model that can be adapted for prenatal clinics, home visiting programs, and health educators. The Baby Basics Toolbox for Change consists of three main components:

- Prenatal health literacy materials: Innovative prenatal health education materials and the health literacy support to assist at-risk expecting women to better understand and access health care for themselves and their children.
- Professional training program: A clear and easy-to-use prenatal health literacy training program for doctors, midwives and nurses, educators, administrators, and clerical staff. This includes

tools and implementation support for health care institutions of varied sizes and structures to welcome their patients, communicate and care for their patients, and engage their patients.

• Coordinated reinforcement: A method for coordinating communitywide interventions across artificial boundaries (for example, health, education, and social services) to provide patient-centered prenatal care. By using the same materials, language, and messaging, the prenatal community—doctors, WIC counselors, home visitors, doulas, and childbirth educators—have a consistent health literacy strategy that supports a communitywide message.

Evaluation

Table 7.1 lists key indicators to be measured in the Jamaica field site by Medical Health Research Associates of New York City.

The Baby Basics Program Model

At a mom's first prenatal appointment at Jamaica Maternity Infant Care she receives, at intake, a copy of *Baby Basics* (or *Hola Bebé*) and a Baby Basics Planner from the clerical staff. The clerical staff will have received Baby Basics implementation training and are able to warmly greet mothers in their native language and introduce the book and program to mothers in an empowering, engaging way. Doctors and midwives also receive brief Baby Basics training. They have learned how to use the new Baby Basics prompt cards and planner to integrate Baby Basics into their visit so that women can look up, write down, and remember the provider's directions. Providers also develop skills in promoting better health literacy in their patients. The nursing and social work staff also receive Baby Basics training. They know how to refer to the *Baby Basics* book when teaching patients and use the same terms and language, and even point to the same pictures and pages when reinforcing prenatal information.

Everyone at the center encourages pregnant women to attend the Baby Basics Moms Club, groups that are held at least once a

Table 7.1. Baby Basics Toolbox Evaluation of Key Indicators.

Some Proposed Measures	Intervention Sites		Nonintervention (Control) Site	
	Baseline	After Implementation	Baseline	After Implementation
Process				
Number of linkages with literacy organizations		X		
Number of *Baby Basics/Hola Bebé* books distributed		X		
Patient satisfaction (as measured by existing patient surveys)	X	X	X	X
Outcome: birth outcomes, birth weight, number of				
nonscheduled visits per patient	X	X	X	X
Number of unnecessary calls to providers with questions	X	X	X	X
Number of missed visits per patient	X	X	X	X
Percentage of pregnant women who smoke during pregnancy	X	X	X	X
Percentage of pregnant women who drink alcohol during pregnancy	X	X	X	X
Percentage of pregnant women who screen positive for depression	X	X	X	X
Percentage of pregnant women who screen positive for anxiety	X	X	X	X
Number of providers trained		X		
Number of women referred to BB Mom's Club, who go to classes, who stay for full classes		X		
Proportion of women returning for postpartum care at MIC center	X	X	X	X
Proportion of women selecting a pediatrician before delivery	X	X	X	X
Mediating				
Presence of other programs and interventions in community	X	X	X	X
Other program enrollment (for example, WIC) for patients studied	X	X	X	X
Readability statistics of existing patient education materials	X		X	

week in the health education room. There, a health educator, who has received Baby Basics training in literacy/ESOL strategies, and in the newly developed Baby Basics Moms Club Curriculum, runs supportive prenatal health literacy groups that foster discussion and group learning. At the Moms Clubs, expectant women meet other pregnant women, learn important prenatal information and how to use *Baby Basics*, and learn about accessing other resources. This club makes the most of the time moms usually spend waiting for their appointment. The waiting room has colorful bookshelves, filled with children's books in English and Spanish lining the walls. Finally, bored older siblings have something to do and learn while waiting for their mother.

Baby Basics is also reinforced in the home. The Baby Basics materials help the home visitor coordinate each woman's entire prenatal experience, from the health center to the home. Baby Basics can be easily used in tandem with whatever curriculum home visitors are already using (such as those created by Nurse Family Partnerships or Healthy Families America). An advantage is that with Baby Basics training, the Baby Basics Moms Club curriculum helps visitors integrate new teaching strategies and health literacy skills into their visits. Also, using the Baby Basics Planner, community health workers are able to see what the doctor or midwife has reviewed with the expectant mother at her previous medical appointment and can build on the visit by reinforcing that information. The home visitor is then able to help her client prepare for her next visit by reviewing tests that will be performed, introducing health vocabulary likely to be encountered, forming and writing down medical questions to ask at the next checkup, and role-playing conversations.

Each of these activities is meant to improve the expectant mother's health literacy and empower her to participate actively in her health care. Quite literally from provider, to educator, to counselor, to home visitor, everyone in a Baby Basics Program is on the same page.

Finally, WIC counselors, HIV coordinators, labor and delivery nurses, and even fatherhood educators are trained to use the Baby Basics materials, providing integrated and reinforced messages to expecting families.

Wrapping Up

This case study demonstrates that conceptualizing, designing, and field-testing materials for target audiences is a collaborative and iterative process that remains open to new information and transforming ideas. By involving members of the health care and adult education communities, as well as members of the target audience, the Baby Basics Program strategically developed a health education program and materials with health literacy principles, specifically fundamental literacy, as a focus. The What to Expect Foundation uses this collaborative model to address its goal of integrating women's fundamental literacy, health literacy, and health. Key strengths and uniqueness of the Baby Basics Program are:

- Clear, readable material, appropriate to audience needs

- Culturally relevant and mindful of readers' contexts

- Emphasis on empowerment of low-literate individuals

- Strategic layout and design

- A health literacy program that asks health care providers as well as patients to adopt new communication strategies

- A distribution plan strategically linked to an education program

- Ongoing evaluation and improvement of the Baby Basics toolbox for change

Exercises

1. Select an existing health education program you are using or know of. Reconstruct as best you can how the program was developed. Identify the amount and kind of target audience input that was used. Does this input seem adequate to you? If yes, explain. If no, describe the types of input you would have recommended.

2. You have been asked to produce a set of consumer health materials and a dissemination plan for a hospital. You are told that once the materials are ready to be printed, you should "try them out" to get reactions from the target audience. Prepare an argument for using a more collaborative approach. Write up a brief outline of how you would get the job done.

8

Anthrax

A Missed Opportunity
to Advance Health Literacy

During late September and early October 2001, massive public attention was focused on the specter of biological terrorism in the United States (see Exhibit 8.1 for a time line). Public discourse about terrorism and bioterrorism dominated content in the traditional mass media, multiplied on the World Wide Web, and topped the agenda around dinner tables and water coolers. The U.S. Postal Service mailed a postcard to every household in the country, while federal and local health departments quickly dusted off, revamped, and expanded emergency plans for potential acts of bioterrorism in the future. In short, the country was trying to rapidly respond to a new threat and struggling to build new understandings of a suddenly changed world.

A tacit agreement, long established between public health officials and the publics they serve, is that timely, accurate, and trustworthy information will be delivered in order to safeguard people's health and well-being. Attempting to prevent overreaction and widespread panic during the anthrax threat, officials needed to give the public and press concrete and understandable information and advice in answer to basic questions:

- What is anthrax?
- Who was at risk?

Text continues on page 170.

Exhibit 8.1. Anthrax in the United States: A Time Line, September to November 2001.

Sept. 18:   Letters postmarked in Trenton, N.J.; sent to *New York Post* and NBC anchor Tom Brokaw. They later test positive for anthrax.

Sept. 22:   Editorial page assistant at *New York Post* who opens letters to the editor notices blister on her finger. Johanna Huden later tests positive for skin form of anthrax, a more treatable form of disease.

Sept. 26:   Maintenance worker at Trenton regional post office in Hamilton, N.J., visits physician to have lesion on arm treated.

Sept. 27:   Teresa Heller, letter carrier at West Trenton post office, develops lesion on her arm.

Sept. 28:   Erin O'Connor, assistant to NBC News anchor Tom Brokaw, notices a lesion.

Sept. 30:   Bob Stevens, photo editor at supermarket tabloid the *Sun* in Boca Raton, Fla., starts to feel ill.

Oct. 1:   Ernesto Blanco, mailroom employee at American Media, publisher of the *Sun*, admitted to hospital with heart problems. O'Connor begins taking Cipro.

Oct. 2:   Stevens admitted to hospital.

Oct. 3:   In New Jersey, Heller is hospitalized and biopsy is performed.

Oct. 4:   Authorities confirm Stevens has inhalation anthrax, most deadly form of disease.
            —Claire Fletcher, assistant to CBS News anchor Dan Rather, begins taking penicillin after visiting doctor. Later, she is tested for anthrax after NBC case becomes public.

Oct. 5:   Stevens dies. First U.S. death from inhaled anthrax since 1976.

Oct. 9:   Letter postmarked in Trenton, N.J., sent to Senate Majority Leader Tom Daschle. It later tests positive for anthrax.

Oct. 12:   Officials announce O'Connor at NBC developed skin
            anthrax after opening letter.

Oct. 14:   Letter containing anthrax opened in Daschle's office.
            Daschle's office quarantined.

Oct. 15:   Officials say infant son of ABC News producer in New York
            developed skin anthrax. The baby, believed to have visited
            the newsroom on September 28, is taking antibiotics and is
            expected to recover.
            —NBC News anchor Brokaw, while holding up a vial of
                pills, says, "In Cipro we trust."

Oct. 16:   Twelve Senate offices closed; hundreds of staffers get tests.

Oct. 17:   Thirty-one people at U.S. Capitol test positive for exposure
            to anthrax, officials say. Later, more complete tests show only
            twenty-eight actually exposed.
            —U.S. House shuts down for testing. Senate stays open two
                more days.
            —New York Governor George Pataki's Manhattan office
                evacuated after test detects presence of anthrax. No one
                tests positive for exposure.

Oct. 18:   Fletcher at CBS tests positive for skin anthrax.
            —The Centers for Disease Control and Prevention hold
                special webcast to teach doctors how to recognize anthrax.
            —New Jersey letter carrier who first got lesion on September
                27 diagnosed with skin anthrax. Another postal worker
                likely had skin anthrax, though tests inconclusive.

Oct. 19:   *New York Post* announces Huden is diagnosed with skin
            anthrax.
            —Another New Jersey postal worker, at Hamilton regional
                office, tests positive for skin anthrax. FBI questions
                residents, businesses on New Jersey mail route of infected
                letter carrier.
            —Anthrax bacteria strains in Florida, New York, and
                Washington may have been from same batch, Homeland
                Security chief Tom Ridge says.

Exhibit 8.1. Anthrax in the United States: A Time Line, September to November 2001, *continued.*

          —U.S. Postal Service sends every American a postcard about handling mail safely.

Oct. 20:   Tests confirm anthrax traces found in mail-bundling machine at House office building a few blocks from the Capitol.

Oct. 21:   Washington postal worker gravely ill with inhalation anthrax; five others sick. Officials close two postal facilities, begin testing thousands of postal employees. Later that night, postal worker Thomas L. Morris Jr. dies.

          —New Jersey health officials say work areas, but not public areas, at Hamilton post office test positive for anthrax spores.

          —Washington postal worker Joseph P. Curseen goes to Maryland hospital complaining of flu-like symptoms. He is sent home.

Oct. 22:   Curseen returns to hospital at 5:45 A.M. by ambulance; dies six hours later of inhalation anthrax. Two other postal workers hospitalized in serious but stable condition.

          —House and Senate reopen; office buildings remain closed.

Oct. 23:   Anthrax found on machinery at military base that sorts mail for White House; all tests at White House itself come back negative. President Bush says: "I don't have anthrax."

          —Officials announce that unidentified New Jersey postal worker at Hamilton office is hospitalized with suspected case of inhalation anthrax.

          —Ernesto Blanco released from hospital after 23 days.

Oct. 24:   Surgeon General David Satcher admits "we were wrong" not to respond more aggressively to tainted mail in Washington. Three new cases of suspected inhalation anthrax announced in Maryland suburbs, all linked to Daschle letter.

Oct. 25:   An employee at the State Department's mail facility is
           hospitalized with anthrax, and the postal service sets up spot
           checks at facilities nationwide.

           —Homeland Security director Ridge says the anthrax in the
             Daschle letter was highly concentrated and made "to be
             more easily absorbed" by its victims.

           —The number of Americans taking antibiotics for possible
             anthrax exposure reaches 10,000.

Oct. 26:   The Supreme Court building is ordered shut down for
           anthrax testing.

           —Postal workers demand the closure of anthrax-tainted
             buildings in New York and Florida, with some union
             officials threatening to sue the postal service.

           —As of October 24: Eleven confirmed and four suspected
             cases (seven inhalation, eight cutaneous). Three letters
             total (two to New York City, one to Washington, D.C.),
             and three deaths.

Nov. 9:   Twenty-two cases of anthrax identified: 10 inhalation, 12
           cutaneous (7 confirmed, 5 suspected). Since October 8,
           32,000 people began antimicrobial prophylaxis to prevent
           infection, and for 5,000 people a 60-day course of antibiotics
           has been recommended.

Nov. 16:   Ninety-four-year-old woman goes to hospital in Oxford,
           Conn., with "fever, cough, weakness, and muscle aches of
           approximately three days' duration."

Nov. 21:   Connecticut patient dies.

Nov. 23:   World Health Organization says 23 cases: 18 confirmed
           (11 inhalation anthrax, 7 cutaneous), 5 suspected. Five
           deaths from inhalation anthrax.

- What were public health officials doing?

- What should the public do?

Public health officials at all levels faced three complex challenges:

- Communicate the complex language of medicine and biology

- Communicate scientific uncertainty and rapidly changing scientific knowledge

- Mediate controversial social equity issues

This case study examines how these complex communication challenges were handled from a health literacy perspective. This approach, focusing on selected sites of communication, reviews elements of the Centers for Disease Control and Prevention web site related to anthrax, selected media coverage from the *New York Times* and network television, and information from the U.S. Postal Service.

The American Public Reacts

The official response to the anthrax threat in the United States can be characterized as a series of attempts to communicate and act with certainty in the face of surprises, scientific uncertainty, and new discoveries. In a variety of official statements, anthrax was first limited to the single case in Florida; then it was not. Later, postal workers were not at risk; then they were. Long after the immediate threat had passed, official statements continued to reflect uncertainty about how spores travel and how many spores are needed for infection. With the first delivery of anthrax, all of the potential problems of forging public communication efforts about a constantly changing, threatening, dreaded risk to human health and security were simultaneously dropped on the health system's doorstep.

Polling data are an indicator of how communication from public health officials and entities was received by the public. Once anthrax hit the news, pollsters immediately began including questions about anthrax. A Gallup poll taken between October 19 and 21, 2001, found that only 13 percent of Americans were "very confident" in the government's ability to prevent additional anthrax exposures. Thirty-eight percent said they were "not too" or "not at all" confident. A Pew Research Center for the People and the Press poll (2001b), conducted between October 10 and 14, found that "about 7 in 10 (69 percent) have some concern over new attacks, and better than half (52 percent) are at least somewhat worried that they or their families could become victims of terrorism."

A poll by the New York Times/CBS News conducted between October 25 and 28 found that 50 percent of the country felt the government was not telling people everything they needed to know about anthrax (Berke & Elder, 2001). A Gallup poll conducted a month later, on November 26 and 27, found that individuals with less formal education were more likely to be worried about exposure to anthrax. Forty-four percent of Americans with a high school education or less were worried compared to 21 percent of those with a college degree (Jones, 2001).

The relationship between formal education and worry about exposure to anthrax is especially relevant to the theme of this book. The Gallup poll results are clear evidence that the public discourse about anthrax did not have the same impact across the population. People with less education (linked to generally lower literacy levels as discussed in Chapters 1 through 3) were twice as likely to be worried about anthrax exposure.

Education level relates not only to how people read and listen but also to what they read and listen to. Literacy and health literacy determine in part how well people understand health risk and related pertinent information. The message to health care communicators is clear: individuals receive and interpret information in their own contexts, through their own ways of understanding, and they draw their own conclusions. The intent of a message does not necessarily equal the impact. If health care communicators want to gain a broader understanding of the impact of their efforts, they need to fully take into account the many contexts of the message, sender, and receiver. (See Chapter 4 for a discussion of contexts.)

The U.S. Postal Service Postcard: A Mixed Success

There was great variation in the complexity of language appearing in the countless messages about the anthrax threat. Perhaps the most widely distributed communication effort was a postcard from the U.S. Postal Service (USPS). According to the USPS (2001), "Every household in America, every rental Post Office box and all military APO and FPO addresses" received a postcard containing information about how to identify and respond to suspicious mail.

The objectives in mailing the card are plainly laid out on the front of the postcard (Exhibit 8.2). The short message from Postmaster General John E. Potter tells readers that the postcard is an attempt to protect customers and employees. Furthermore, the postal service wanted to leave readers with a sense that there was something they could do in response to the risk of anthrax exposure. In fact, the postmaster explicitly informed Americans, "We need your help."

The central goal of the postcard is to provide specific advice and action steps for a broad range of individuals at all literacy levels who are concerned about their own risk and seeking concrete responses to the risk. Although the postcard seems to be a series of brief, easy-to-follow steps, crucial messages remain complex and beyond the reading level of nearly half the U.S. population.

Vocabulary

All of the following examples on the postcard contain unnecessarily difficult vocabulary:

Exhibit 8.2. USPS Postcard Regarding Suspicious Mail.

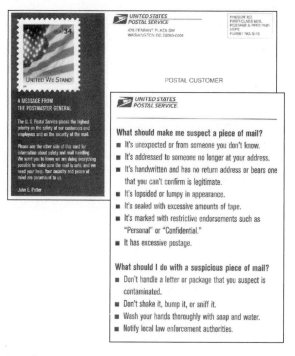

Source: http://www.usps.gov/news/2001/press/mailsecurity/postcard.htm.

"It's sealed with excessive amount of tape." "Excessive" is approximately a ninth-grade-level word. *Suggested revision for better understanding:* "It's wrapped in too much tape."

"It's marked with restrictive endorsements such as 'personal' or 'Confidential.'" *Suggested revision for better understanding:* "It has the words 'Personal' and 'Confidential' on it."

"It has excessive postage." *Suggested revision for better understanding:* "It has a lot of postage on it."

Sentences

The card contains examples of easy-to-read and hard-to-read language. The seven phrases describing suspicious mail are generally simple, clear, and printed in a large and easy-to-read font. Perhaps the most difficult linguistic concept on the rear of the postcard, where most of the information and action steps are clearly bulleted, is the phrase "restrictive endorsements." That phrase is immediately unpacked with examples of "personal" or "confidential," but that does not fully overcome the initial barrier to readers created by difficult language.

Using a consistent grammatical construction for each bulleted item is a good strategy and aids readability. However, the readability of the card is not at a consistent fifth-grade reading level, so there are a number of hard-to-read sentences—for example:

- "It's unexpected or from someone you don't know."

This sentence structure is missing necessary elements. The referent ("piece of mail") is deleted, and the verb ("it comes from/is from") does not appear in the sentence. The reader has to infer the meaning from the general context. A *solution:* "The mail is not expected, or it comes from someone you do not know."

- "It's addressed to someone no longer at your address."

This is another example of a deleted construction. A *solution:* "The mail is for someone who does not live at your address."

- "It's handwritten and has no return address or bears one that you can't confirm is legitimate."

The idea of a "legitimate address" is not a simple one, and the postcard provides no definition or clue as to what is or is not a legitimate address. Therefore, this concept is insufficiently communicated in no small part due to its somewhat amorphous nature. A *solution:* "The mail is handwritten and has no return address. If there is a return address, you cannot tell if it is a real address."

- "It's lopsided or lumpy in appearance."

Because "lopsided" and "lumpy" may not be familiar reading words, readers need clues that will help them predict the meaning of these words. A *solution:* "The mail looks or feels lumpy or lopsided."

The phrases describing what could be suspect mail are followed by a short list of action steps to be taken if an individual considers a piece of mail suspicious (see Exhibit 8.2). The suggested actions are both precautionary and responsive steps that attempt to create a verbal road map to safety for the millions of Americans who received the post card. However, alternative language choices could have improved readability. For example, the list could be revised in this way:

- If you think a piece of mail is suspicious or may be not safe:

  Do NOT touch the letter or package.

  Do NOT shake the letter or package.

  Do NOT bang, bump, or drop the letter or package.

  Wash your hands very well with soap and water.

  Call the police right away.

Seeking Anthrax Answers on the Internet

There is a tremendous amount of health-related information on the internet. Over 100,000 health-related sites (Eysenbach et al., 1999) are available, and almost 100 million Americans regularly go online for health information. One estimate is that over 34 percent of online activity is a search for information about health services or practices (National Telecommunications and Information Administration, 2004). Many individuals who searched for answers about anthrax used the Internet, and many of those no doubt saw information drawn from the Centers for Disease Control and Prevention (CDC).

The CDC was a primary source of information from the U.S. government during the anthrax threat. At the time, a link on the CDC home page (2002b), "Terrorism and Public Health—Info for Partners, Professionals and the Public," led to a definition of anthrax written at the college and postcollege level that is quite inaccessible due to complex vocabulary and embedded compound and complex sentences (Exhibit 8.3).

In contrast to the postal service's mass mailing, the definition of anthrax the CDC offers is uniformly complex in vocabulary and

Exhibit 8.3. CDC Web Site Definition of Anthrax.

Definition

What is anthrax?

Bacillus anthracis, the etiologic agent of anthrax, is a large, gram-positive, non-motile, spore-forming bacterial rod. The three virulence factors of B. *anthracis* are edema toxin, lethal toxin and a capsular antigen. Human anthrax has three major clinical forms: cutaneous, inhalation, and gastrointestinal. If left untreated, anthrax in all forms can lead to septicemia and death.

What is the case definition for anthrax?

A confirmed case of anthrax is defined as

1. a clinically compatible case of cutaneous, inhalational, or gastrointestinal illness that is laboratory-confirmed by isolation of B. *anthracis* from an affected tissue or site, or
2. a clinically compatible case of cutaneous, inhalational, or gastrointestinal disease with other laboratory evidence of B. *anthracis* infection based on at least two supportive laboratory tests.

Source: http://www.bt.cdc.gov/DocumentsApp/FAQAnthrax.asp.

sentence structure. For example, the first two sentences—"*Bacillus anthracis*, the etiologic agent of anthrax, is a large, gram-positive, non-motile, spore-forming bacterial rod. The three virulence factors of B. *anthracis* are edema toxin, lethal toxin and a capsular antigen"—are readable with comprehension only for those with some medical training.

The third sentence, "Human anthrax has three major clinical forms: cutaneous, inhalation, and gastrointestinal," contains a smattering of more communicative elements but then runs into a roadblock when assuming the reader understands the embedded concept of a "clinical form." Even readers with a high enough level of literacy to understand the words *cutaneous, inhalation,* and *gastrointestinal* may not have a level of health literacy equal to that concept; only through backward detective work can they cobble together a concept of what "clinical form" means.

With the exception of the words *anthrax* and *death,* most readers would not understand this definition. When a text is hard to read, readers will generally persist, rearranging the text to make some meaning, even if it is not the text's intended meaning. For example, a frequently used reading strategy of skipping and guessing would likely lead readers of the fourth sentence to the following reconstructed meaning: "If left untreated, anthrax in all forms can lead to septicemia and death."

Although there were excellent, easy-to-read examples of media and government messages during the anthrax threat, it is often more instructional to focus on where communication was difficult or less successful. This section of the CDC web site was one of those cases. Within the domain of fundamental literacy, the complex language does not meet basic needs of most readers: it does not use shared, common language. This definition by the CDC could actually do harm by misinforming or turning citizens to other, perhaps less reliable sources of information.

Scientific Uncertainty: A Consistent Challenge

Complexity generally creates uncertainty. Inherent in bioterrorism is a dual potential for mass destruction (death and illness) and mass disruption (fear, panic, and mistrust of official sources). Without uncertainty, there would be less disruption. In the case of anthrax-tainted letters in the United States, disruption occurred on a larger scale than destruction.

Two critical areas of uncertainty contributed to the potential for broad social disruption during the anthrax threat. First, there was uncertainty about what action a bioterrorist would next take. Second, there were scientific uncertainties about anthrax itself.

Bioterrorism, however, ripped open the "black box" of knowledge about anthrax (Latour, 1987). Bioterrorism brought into full public display the scientific uncertainty about the amount of spores that can cause inhalation anthrax; the ability of anthrax to cross-contaminate other pieces of mail, buildings, and processing machinery; and the likelihood of secondary aerosolization of anthrax spores. Public health officials needed to address these uncertainties to successfully answer the public's questions and dispel unwarranted fears that potentially could lead to greater social disruption. However, at times the science was not at hand to answer those questions even though anthrax was first identified over 100 years ago and served as the basis for the development of Koch's Postulates in 1890, which set the criteria still in use today for judging whether a given bacterium is the cause of a given disease.

Anthony Fauci, director of the National Institute of Allergy and Infectious Diseases of the National Institutes of Health, was later described in *U.S. News and World Report* as "the nation's go-to guy when it comes to explaining the new facts of life with bioterrorism" (Shute, 2002, p. 32). When asked by Katie Couric on NBC's *Today* show on October 15, 2001, what the response would be for postal workers if anthrax spores were found in their facility, Fauci described the scientific process as it was being applied to determining the response to anthrax at various postal facilities in understandable terms. He attempted to improve the science literacy of the viewers.

> As you know, this is a work in progress because it is still not certain, as we have not heard from the CDC, as to whether or not there are more of these letters in addition to the Daschle letter [referring to a letter sent to Senator Tom Daschle containing anthrax spores]. But let's just assume, for example, that there is a letter that has some contamination. The primary facility in Washington, D.C., is the Brentwood facility that is clearly contaminated, so anyone who is in that facility and han-

dling bulk mail needs to be treated. . . . There has already
been documentation that people have gotten inhalation
anthrax from secondary facilities. So the assumption is
that if one is contaminated they might all be contaminated. Therefore, preemptively, people are being given
antibiotics while their facility is being swept for the
evidence of there being contamination. If it is contaminated, then you continue the antibiotics. If it isn't,
then that is when you have heard about giving people
10 days just to make sure they are covered. Then if the
tests come back that in fact their particular facility is
negative—there has been no contamination—then you
can withdraw. That is the general philosophy that has
been put forth.

Fauci addressed the concept that scientific and medical understandings are works in progress—a complex notion for a citizenry
more accustomed to perceiving science as a source of distinct
answers and universal truths (Nelkin, 1987; Friedman, Dunwoody,
& Rogers, 1999; Gregory & Miller, 1998). He also attempted
to explain the contingencies of treatment for postal workers depending on the evidence of exposure and the stance toward risk that
was taken.

Fauci's message left viewers with the assurance that not only was
there a specific response to a specific situation, but that there was a
general philosophy in place. He accomplished all this in a language
in which the most complex phrases were notions of "contamination,"
"documentation," and "secondary facilities." If the sort of communication he delivered was the norm rather than the exception, public
health literacy could have clearly benefited.

Another example of a concept far less successfully communicated was the concept of appropriate use of antibiotics. Public
opinion polls during the anthrax threat found that between 3 and
6 percent of the public reported obtaining a prescription for an

antibiotic (Blendon, Benson, DesRoches, & Herrmann, 2001). As a percentage, that seems a relatively modest reaction, but in real numbers, 3 percent of the U.S. population is over 8 million people. The core dilemma for individuals was the decision between what was perceived as a personal protective measure (taking antibiotics) or maintaining concern about a potential public health threat many were unaware or poorly informed of (antibiotic resistance).

On that same episode of the *Today* show, replying to Couric's question about the possibility of treating the entire U.S. population with antibiotics, Fauci said, "That, in and of itself, if done has a potential for danger from the antibiotics themselves that might actually even eclipse what we are talking about right now." While Fauci took great pains to communicate the nature of uncertainty, he was lacking in a complete explanation. In most other cases, the lack of complete explanation resulted in conflicting statements about what people could do in order to protect themselves during the anthrax threat.

On a basic level, it was never well explained why each American should not universally take an antibiotic like ciprofloxacin (Cipro) other than through scare-fueling discussions about the shortage of the antibiotic. Antibiotic resistance is an example of a moment when individuals can take actions to protect themselves, but those actions can eventually be harmful to themselves and others. What was common knowledge to public health officials and health providers was not equally shared by the American public. The following text box presents one way to explain antibiotic resistance.

Wrapping Up

In this chapter, we have examined fundamental health literacy challenges in greater detail. In particular, we have seen that difficult language without definition and explanation, complex sentence structure, assumed knowledge, and scientific uncertainty are among

Antibiotic Resistance

Why You Don't Want to Take Antibiotics When You Don't Need Them

The news media have talked a lot about using antibiotics like Cipro during this anthrax outbreak. It is very important to understand that while antibiotics are effective, they can create problems when they are not used correctly. Public health officials are worried about the problem of antibiotic resistance, when antibiotics no longer kill the bacteria.

What Causes Antibiotic Resistance?

Bacteria, like anthrax, group in colonies. Each bacterium in a colony is not the same. Some die quickly when exposed to an antibiotic. Others do not die quickly; they are resistant to the antibiotic. The bacteria that survive reproduce, and their offspring inherit their resistance. Eventually, only the most resistant bacteria survive. Each generation of bacteria can build up resistance so the antibiotic does not work anymore. When resistant bacteria infect a person, that person will not respond to antibiotic treatment. This often has serious or fatal results.

Scientists have studied antibiotic treatment for over 50 years. They have seen this problem of antibiotic resistance when treating many diseases, such as tuberculosis, streptococcal infections, and venereal diseases.

So it is very important that people take antibiotics only when needed and exactly as they are instructed. If too many people take antibiotics when they do not need them, antibiotic resistance increases. If antibiotic resistance increases, antibiotics will not work when we really need them. This is an important public health problem you can do something about.

the important issues that must be addressed. We explored several key issues faced by health communicators and several methods of response during the 2001 anthrax threat. Although we have focused on fundamental health literacy, we have also referred to instances where scientific and civic literacy are necessary to better comprehend the anthrax threat.

Exercises

1. Research and craft a definition of anthrax. Then, using that definition and those of your classmates as the raw material, try to come to agreement (or consensus) on a best definition for anthrax. (Note to instructors: Introduce the problems of coming to scientific consensus and the multiple pressures and agendas agencies like the CDC face when creating communication pieces.)

2. Given that the specter of bioterrorism remains a sad reality, break the class up into groups representing the CDC, the White House, and the National Institutes of Health, a state department of health, and a local mayor. Try to develop a plan to respond to a threat of bioterrorism. How are the agendas in conflict or agreement? What should or should not be incorporated into such a plan?

3. Using a database like Lexis-Nexis, find examples of media coverage of the anthrax threat from a variety of newspapers around the United States and internationally. Examine the examples for differences in content, tone, and reading level. Discuss the similarities and differences found.

9

Genomics and Health Literacy

During the past few centuries, science has produced the foundations of knowledge and technology for at least two revolutions in the way people, particularly in high-income countries like the United States, go about their daily affairs and make sense of the world. One of those revolutions is caused by the computer and internet, discussed in Chapter 6. The second is often called genomics.

Genomics is a catch-all term representing the many different forms of knowledge, application, and scientific investigation related to the structure and function of DNA (deoxyribonucleic acid). The term has been used to refer to academic disciplines, business ventures, clinical practices, and even folk ideas of heredity.

Why Genomics?

We can imagine a healthy individual living in an equally healthy family in a society that never experiences or witnesses illness. In such a place, through some stroke of magic, no one needs health literacy skills or everyone has unimaginably high levels of high literacy. In such a place, no one is left wondering why illness struck this friend and not another. In such a place, no one tests their future children's genetic makeup for diseases like Down syndrome or Huntington's chorea. However, we can only imagine such a place, as it certainly does not exist. Health literacy is a necessity to keep up with the continuing advances in the scientific understandings of health and medical practice. Genomics is at the cutting edge of that knowledge.

On an almost daily basis, we read or hear about the discovery of genes "for" breast cancer, or encounter folklore about the genetic basis of race, or simply hear someone say, "It's genetic." A small handful of us read textbooks with titles like *Polymerase Chain Reaction and Other Methods for In Vitro DNA Amplifications*, but all of us have cells, chromosomes, genes, and DNA. Physicians and patients, counselors and clients, politicians and voters, journalists and audiences are all encountering some fundamental notions of genomics in their day-to-day lives. Examples include the following:

- James Watson, Nobel Prize winner for the discovery of the double-helix structure of DNA, claimed that "a more important set of instruction books will never be found by human beings. When finally interpreted, the genetic messages encoded within our DNA molecules will provide the ultimate answers to the chemical underpinnings of human existence" (Watson, 1990, p. 44). Watson was also quoted in *Time* magazine as saying, "We used to think our fate was in the stars. Now we know, in large measure, our fate is in our genes" (Jaroff, 1989, p. 67).

- The first person freed from death row by DNA evidence, Kirk Bloodsworth, was quoted in the *New York Times*: "To me, DNA is like the silver bullet to the werewolf of injustice" ("A Revolution at 50," 2003, p. F5).

- On the announcement of the mapping, albeit a rough draft, of the human genome, U.S. President Bill Clinton said, "Today we are learning the language in which God created life" (Wade, 2000, p. A1).

The complexity of genomics presents challenges not only for members of the public but also for health care providers. For example, despite wide agreement on the important potential of this area of scientific knowledge, Francis Collins, director of the National Human Genome Research Institute of the National Institutes of Health, cautions, "Doctors and other health professionals are not yet prepared to inform patients about the appropriate applications of genetic tests or to provide basic genetic education and counseling as more genetic tests and technologies become available" (Collins & Bochm, 1999, p. 48). Health care providers are far from alone, as very few individuals have a high level of health literacy in regard to genomics. If even a fraction of the potential impact of mapping the human genome is realized, everyone should have some basic familiarity with what DNA is, how it works, and what that means.

However, scientists and medical specialists are often so focused on their particular microcosm of expertise that they lose sight of the larger picture. Generalists and family practitioners are challenged to keep up with the constant production of new knowledge about genomics. Journalists tend to follow the newsworthy story of the day, often missing individual differences or how each piece of new scientific knowledge does or does not fit into a larger meaning or into individual lives. As a result, the public receives fragmented bits and pieces of information about DNA, genetics, chromosomes, and the promise of large-scale scientific enterprises from a wide variety of uncoordinated, and often unreliable, sources.

Given that context and the potential of genomics, it is no surprise that there are many large and ongoing efforts to educate the public about genomics. Examples exist around the world, ranging from a book, *Your Genes, Your Choices* (Baker, 1999), created and published by the American Association for the Advancement of Science in an attempt to educate low-literate readers about genetics and the Human Genome Project, to the Public Understanding of Biotechnology initiative sponsored by the government of South Africa.

It remains difficult to measure and describe the effects of such efforts, although there is at least a decade of effort measuring public understanding of science. The underlying hypothesis of many of those efforts is that the more scientifically literate a person is, the more positive that person will feel about science and the greater trust that person will place in scientists and the products of science. However, that has not always the case (Pardo & Calvo, 2002).

For example, a study in Finland on the relationship between knowledge of and attitudes toward genetic testing found that those with the lowest level of knowledge had the most difficulty in taking a position in response to attitude statements in the survey. However, a higher level of understanding of genetics did not predict unequivocal support or enthusiasm for genetic testing. In fact, the researchers found that although greater genetics literacy is associated with a higher level of acceptance, it is also associated with greater levels of suspicion and uncertainty (Jallinoja & Aro, 2000).

The discussions about genomics reflect every aspect of health literacy. The rich and complex interplay of fundamental, scientific, civic, and cultural domains quickly rises to the surface when we talk about one of the most fundamental elements of life. Thus, as a case study, genomics demonstrates the utility of our model of health literacy not only for addressing individuals with low health literacy, but also as an aid for those needing to communicate complicated cutting-edge understandings of our bodies and health.

In this chapter, we explore the challenges and demands on an individual's health literacy within the discourse about genomics. We pay particular attention to the scientific literacy domain of health literacy. After briefly exploring shifts in how genomics has been discussed over time, we focus on two elements of communication frequently used to explain aspects of genomics: the use of metaphor and the use of proportions.

Understanding and Misunderstanding Genomics: A Review

In six surveys of the public understanding of science in the United States between 1988 and 1999, an average of only 19.5 percent responded correctly to the open-ended question, "What is DNA?"

Scientific Literacy

We define scientific literacy as the level of competence with physical and natural sciences, including the scientific process and technology, and encompassing:

- Knowledge of fundamental science concepts

- An ability to comprehend technical complexity

- An understanding of technology

- An understanding of scientific uncertainty and that rapid change in the accepted science is possible

Understanding medical science is just one component of health literacy. Our model of health literacy reflects how that understanding is incorporated into individual decision making.

(Miller & Kimmel, 2001). Despite that apparent low level of understanding, consider how often you hear the phrases, "It's genetic" or "It must be in her genes."

In another example, 80 percent of 220 women surveyed while going for a routine medical visit in Alabama incorrectly believed that 1 in 10 women has an altered breast cancer gene. Nearly three-fourths of the women incorrectly believed that half of all breast cancer cases occur in women who have an altered breast cancer gene (Donovan & Tucker, 2000). The current scientific understanding is that fewer than 10 percent of all breast cancer cases are associated with the "breast cancer genes" BRCA1 and BRCA2. Despite that, consider how often you have seen a newspaper or magazine

Folklore: What Causes Birth Defects and Genetic Disorders?

Many individuals and cultures have attributed birth defects or genetic disorders to an experience the mother had during pregnancy, higher beings or supernatural powers, food, the moon, or the evil eye. Examples include beliefs in some cultures that (Cohen, Fine & Pergament, 1998):

- A cleft lip is caused by looking at or eating a rabbit—hence, the name *harelip*.

- A child will be born with a birth defect if a pregnant woman takes pity on or mocks an affected individual.

- A family is "given" a child with a disorder as a punishment from God for parental sin.

- The "evil eye," an eye or glance held capable of inflicting harm, is a force that determines bad fortune, including birth defects.

- The moon, specifically a lunar eclipse, is a cause of cleft lip or palate.

- Certain foods are to blame. For example, some believe spina bifida can result from eating potato eyes during pregnancy or that chili peppers can cause blindness in the fetus.

- Microcephaly or anencephaly results when the mother looks at a monkey during the pregnancy.

These populist misconceptions create the mental frameworks from which many people may begin to judge scientific understandings of the human genome and the structure and functions of DNA.

headline or heard a television news personality exclaim, "The breast cancer gene has been found" or, more misleading yet, "Genes predict behavior." It is no surprise that so many of the women participating in the Alabama study gave incorrect responses. Clearly, misperceptions, misunderstandings, and plain falsehoods about DNA, genes, and the scientific process are common.

Indications are that the public understands very little about DNA, protein synthesis, or genes. In many instances, low levels of scientific literacy may not be associated with a negative outcome. In other instances, it is possible that individuals hold a very high level of understanding about genomics without being able to correctly wield the jargon of the field as requested in surveys of the public's understanding. However, there are clearly instances when a level of understanding is critical to individual and public health. In the next section, we discuss how the understanding of genes and DNA has changed through time and the implications of that history to current understanding.

The Gene: A Brief History
of Metaphors and Misunderstandings

Whether enlightening, misleading, productive, dangerous, or simply incorrect, some notion of a "gene" being related to the passing down of traits from grandparents to parents to self has existed for centuries in science as well as in indigenous knowledge and popular beliefs.

During the early decades of the twentieth century, a mixture of science and popular culture called eugenics created a dark cloud over public and private discourse about inheritance and genomics. Eugenics fueled notions of genetic superiority that were employed to substantiate the atrocious actions of Nazi Germany. Adolf Hitler, however, was not alone in misunderstanding and misapplying what little was known about genes. The United States was the site of at least 30,000 forced sterilizations of individuals, more of whom were women than men and many of whom were labeled "feeble-minded." The U.S. government also passed restrictive immigration laws under the broad banner of eugenics to improve the "stock" of the American public.

Fortunately, eugenics is only one of many influences in the evolution of public understanding of the genome and its capabilities. Celeste Michelle Condit has documented shifts in popular discourse

---

Fitter Families Competitions: Popularizing Eugenics

The first Fitter Family Contest was held at the Kansas State Free Fair in 1920, emerging from roots in "better baby" contests that had occurred (and still do) at state fairs (Exhibit 9.1). With support from the American Eugenics Society, the contests were held at numerous fairs throughout the United States during the 1920s. According to the Eugenics Archive of the Dolan DNA Learning Center at Cold Spring Harbor laboratory, "At most contests, competitors submitted an Abridged Record of Family Traits, and a team of medical doctors performed psychological and physical exams on family members. Each family member was given an overall letter grade of eugenic health, and the family with the highest grade average was awarded a silver trophy. Trophies were typically awarded in three family categories: small (1 child), medium (2–4 children), and large (5 or more children). All contestants with a B+ or better received bronze medals bearing the inscription, 'Yea, I have a goodly heritage.' As expected, the Fitter Families Contest mirrored the eugenics movement itself; winners were invariably white with northern and western European heritage" (Dolan, 2003, p. 1).

about genetics through time by analyzing magazines, newspapers, television programs, and the *Congressional Record* (Condit, 1999). We can trace that discourse beginning with an early discussion of classical eugenics from roughly 1900 to 1935 when the primary metaphor of genomics was drawn from stock breeding, as captured in phrases such as "Breeding better men."

As both the scientific and political enterprises under the banner of eugenics receded, the public dialogue shifted from discussions of controlling genes to notions of genes controlling individuals. Talk about superior genetics was replaced with discussions of "normal" versus "abnormal."

**Exhibit 9.1. Fitter Family Examining Staff
with Winning Family, Kansas State Free Fair, Topeka, 1920.**

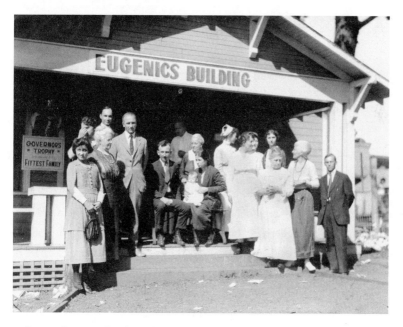

Source: Reprinted with permission, www.eugenicsarchive.org.

The discovery of the structure of DNA in 1953 led to the next shift in how people understood and talked about genomics. During this phase, the notion of DNA working as a code became a dominant metaphor. Today we still often encounter such metaphors in expressions like "genetic code" and the effort to "break the code." Extending this metaphor, parts of the structure of DNA were often referred to as "letters" and groups of them spelled out "words."

The Code Metaphor: An Example

In the question-and-answer section of a brochure produced in 2001 by the U.S. government, "Genes and Populations," a question posed is: "What's involved in this sort of genetics research study?"

The answer reads: "Your body is made up of individual units called cells. Your DNA (your personal genetic code) is tucked inside each of your cells. If you agree to participate in a genetics research study, scientists will collect a small sample of your cells in order to read this code. . . . Scientists will study the DNA from these samples and, through laboratory techniques, they will read the spellings of your genes" (National Institute of General Medical Sciences, 2001, p. 5).

According to Condit, the 1980s and 1990s saw the rise of a "blueprint" metaphor for DNA and a shift in emphasis toward personal health and a growing awareness of the ethical, legal, and social issues related to genomics. Biotechnology ventures began to boom, as did the publicly funded Human Genome Project, which brought genomics out of obscure medical laboratories and into Wall Street's investment portfolios and, eventually, farmers' fields and family dinner tables. The blueprint metaphor neatly aligns with the spirit of business and entrepreneurship that accompanied a shift in much of the press coverage of genomics from the health section to the business section.

The discourse, however, is continually shifting. In the past few years, "The gene metamorphosed into the 'genome', genetics into 'genomics', and the geneticist became an amalgam of a molecular biologist and a computer scientist" (Dijk, 1998, p. 120). The language used to describe genomics, particularly the metaphors, is becoming more complex. Currently, metaphors used often refer to a complex network or a computer program that scientists can map.

How Metaphors Work: A Quick Primer

Metaphors are everywhere in language. Some estimate that people use around five metaphors during every minute of speaking (Glucksberg, 1989). There are generally three reasons people use metaphors when communicating (Gibbs, 1996):

- To express ideas difficult to convey using literal language

- To communicate more succinctly than literal language allows

- To deliver a richer, more vivid understanding than would result from literal language

A metaphor's effect occurs from the comparison of two things: the subject (the thing being described) and the predicate of the metaphor (the thing the subject is being compared to). For example, in the classic metaphoric phrase, "Love is like a red, red rose," the subject is love and the predicate is "a red, red, rose." In a more contemporary example, "That's cool," *that* is the subject, and *cool* is the predicate.

A challenge arises because speakers and writers of metaphor inherently deliver both a literal and an intended meaning (Searle,

1993). For example, literally that love *is* a red, red rose, which makes no sense. The intended meaning is that love has qualities of a red, red rose, leaving it open to interpretation whether love is the color, the petals, the scent, or the thorns. Thus, the interpretation of metaphors is often inexact or grounded in different contexts to produce different meaning. As a result, metaphors are subject to varying interpretations by the audience, and those interpretations will change with varying health literacy skills.

Many metaphors are ingrained into the way we look at the world. For example, "He finally lost his long battle with cancer," reflects a core metaphor of illness as an enemy or invader. Metaphors are so ingrained into our use of language that communicating without metaphors is not only stilted and unnatural, it would place a great burden on both the language and the communicators to find precise enough language to make good meaning. Eliminating metaphors would require more, longer, and more complicated messages, increasing the literacy burden on senders and receivers of messages alike. Thus, another challenge to the use of metaphor is aligning new metaphors with previously held understandings. That challenge is very real using metaphors to communicate complex scientific understandings, such as genomics.

Using Metaphors to Communicate Complex Science

Metaphors are often used to communicate complex science such as genomics. For those with low literacy and low health literacy, the use of metaphor can, in the best instances, improve understanding, but it can also create a barrier to understanding when used improperly.

When metaphors are used to communicate complex science to a nonscientific public, the subject of a metaphor is often the less commonly encountered concept, and the predicate of a metaphor is often the more common of the two concepts. In these cases, metaphors are employed to transform the unusual, science, into the usual example drawn from common life experience. For example,

The Many Metaphors for DNA and Genes

- "A code"
- "A library"
- "A language"
- "A blueprint"
- "A director"
- "Like literature"
- "Selfish"
- "A fundamental building block"
- "An instruction manual for all life"
- "A diary"
- "An alphabet"
- "The silver bullet to the werewolf of injustice"
- "Our fate"
- "The language in which God created life"
- "Like Coca-Cola"
- "A semiconductor"
- "Information storage module"
- "A self-contained macrosystem of control"
- "The molecule of life"
- "A long fiber, like a hair, only thinner and longer (except for Crystal Gayle's hair)"
- "Read-only memory"
- "Life—the rest is just details"

the metaphorical phrase "DNA is like a library" attempts to use the more familiar idea of a library to help explain the more uncommon and complex notion of DNA.

Jonathon Marks (2002) argues that scientists use the metaphors the way they do because it is in their best interests not to dispute popular wisdom, or folk ideologies, because they rely on popular support for funding. We find that to be an interesting but not altogether proven argument as it is equally likely that scientists, who are generally not trained in communication skills or language use, are simply struggling to find language they are comfortable with that also makes some sense to nonscientists.

Another caution of the use of metaphors, specifically in relation to the multibillion dollar effort of the Human Genome Project, comes from Thomas Fogle, who argues the metaphors often used tend to imply that biology determines outcomes and can lead to false expectations (Fogle, 1995).

Nobel prize winner and president of the California Institute of Technology David Baltimore says this about his scientific colleagues' attempts to use metaphor to explain DNA: "They have all decided that the real meaning of this achievement is so wrapped up in technical detail that the only way to convey the truth is through metaphor. So they tell the world that the genome is like a book, with words, sentences, and chapters. Or they say that it is the periodic table for biologists, assuming that laypeople will have heard of this key organizing principle of chemistry. But these and other metaphoric links miss the real story. The genome is like no other object that science has elucidated" (Baltimore, n.d.).

One challenge to the use of metaphor to communicate science lies in the multiple interpretations that metaphors allow. For example, while trying to rely on a metaphor as an explanatory device, George Annas, a professor of health law at Boston University, was trapped within the multiple interpretations of the metaphor he employed during an interview airing on a National Public Radio (NPR) program, *The DNA Files*, produced by SoundVision Productions. Annas said,

Mel Gibson in Each of Our Cells?

With their sole reliance on sound, radio journalists face one of the greatest challenges in mass media communication. During a segment of *The DNA Files*, produced by SoundVision Productions and broadcast on NPR, host John Hockenberry faced that challenge when interviewing Nancy Wexler, a professor of medicine and genetics. Following is the exchange as journalist and scientist grappled with the challenge:

HOCKENBERRY: Each cell in our body, and there are trillions of them in there, contains a copy of our body's genetic information.

WEXLER: If you unroll that genetic information and then you stand it end to end, it's going to be about the length of a six-feet-tall man.

HOCKENBERRY: Professor Nancy Wexler of Columbia University in New York is an expert on genetic disease. She says, imagine that all your genetic information is as tall as, say, the actor Mel Gibson.

WEXLER: If you have Mel Gibson rolled up in every cell and you unroll Mel Gibson, and then you stretch a trillion Mel Gibsons end to end, that's just the amount of DNA one person has in one person's body.

Consider the challenge a person with low literacy skills, tuning in and out while driving to work, would have with this dialogue. High- and low-literate individuals alike could likely gather the impression that they have the same DNA as Mel Gibson or that Mel Gibson actually is in their DNA.

"The DNA molecule, I think, can be analogized to a diary. It's not a diary in the sense that you write things down when you're young that you're going to read about when you're old. But it's a diary in the sense that it's very private information that informs your younger self about your aging self, if you will. It's your diary" (DNA Files, 1998, p. 15). To take Annas literally, as individuals with low health literacy may very well do when challenged to make any meaning, DNA both is and is not a diary. So what is it then?

While using metaphors to communicate science is generally a well-intentioned effort to reduce uncertainty and complexity by making the unusual seem familiar, the use of metaphor can have the opposite result. In health, such misunderstandings between a provider and a patient can create negative outcomes such as poor compliance or a failure to seek proper care. While a metaphor is a powerful component of language, it should be used with care and double-checked to make sure that the intended meaning is actually the meaning people receive.

Probabilities and Percentages: Problems in Communicating Genomics and Risk

Numbers are the lifeblood of quantitative methods in science. Numbers communicate authority and a sense of concrete exactness. Culturally, we place a high value on the ability to quantify and the ability to deal with complex mathematics and statistical calculations, that is, on the ability to use numbers. However, just as is the case with metaphoric language, the use of numbers to explain complex scientific findings can be as misleading as it can be informative.

In particular, there is an increasing use of genetic screenings in everyday health care that among many other effects increases the use of numbers, particularly proportions, as a means of explaining health care options. In this section we address some of the difficulties that approach creates for individuals with low health literacy.

Genetic screenings generally deliver a probability rather than a certainty. The probability, expressed in numbers, tends to obscure the multiple layers of complex and abstract scientific theories, methods, and findings that produced the numbers communicated. In many cases, the information communicated about the results of a genetic screening is a probability of some negative outcome. That information begins a complex task of assessing risk. Despite the wishes of many in the scientific and medical field, the assessment of risk inherently incorporates the many ethical, legal, and social implications of genomic technologies. The health decision, then, is certainly more complex than simply the appropriate assessment of a probability. Examples of such probabilities include:

"Your children will have a one in four chance of being . . ."

"Your children will have a 25 percent likelihood of developing . . ."

More rarely the opposite framing will be used, for example:

"Your children have a 75 percent chance of not developing . . ."

Medicine, and the vast array of technology now in place, is so focused on identifying illness or the potential for ill health that the positive framing of such results is not considered relevant very often except in those cases when doctors get to deliver good news. Sole reliance on a negative frame certainly does nothing to mitigate the psychological impact on patients when receiving the results of genetic screenings. In turn, that frame lessens the likelihood that an individual will correctly process the complex information they receive at such moments.

In this section, we explore several issues:

- The health literacy challenges presented by relying on proportions to explain complex scientific evidence

- How fully patients and providers understand proportions

- If an expert assessment of risk is the only assessment of risk

- Why patients and the public may make decisions that do not make sense to experts

In a classic example of how probabilities are commonly misunderstood, Ruth Hubbard and Elijah Wald break down the rather well-publicized statistic that a woman's chance of getting breast cancer in the United States is one in nine (Hubbard & Wald, 1993). The equally classic and misleading graphic that often accompanies such declarations is an outline of nine women, one of them in a different shade indicating the odds ratio in action: never changing and blind to any other differences between individuals such as lifestyle-based risk factors and genetic makeup. Hubbard and Wald correctly point out that "even for older women, the probabilities at any one time never get nearly as high as 1 in 9" (p. 86). That odds ratio is the cumulative probability over all women's life spans and is never equal to the possibility at any single moment in any single woman's life. However, many people, certainly those with low fundamental literacy and numeracy skills, interpret such probabilities as indicating their chance at every moment during their life and as a chance that remains equal throughout life.

Hubbard and Wald illustrate this poor communication practice by breaking down the incidence of breast cancer for a hypothetical group of 100 women in 10-year increments across 8 decades. During each of the 10-year periods between the ages of 30 to 40 and the ages of 40 to 50, 1 woman will develop breast cancer (1 in 100); between ages 50 and 60, 2 of the 100 women will develop breast cancer (1 in 50). Between ages 60 and 70, 10 of the women have died for various reasons, and 2 of the remaining 90 will develop breast cancer (1 in 45). The age-relevant proportions proceed in a similar fashion so that during any single decade, the odds of 1 of those original 100 women developing breast cancer never exceed 1 in 30. Over an 8-decade span, however, the cumulative probability is roughly 1 in 9.

That is not to say the one-in-nine figure should never be used because there are valid and useful contexts for using such a statistic. The decision on what statistic to use should hinge on the important factors of audience, context, and goals of the health communicator. For example, the one-in-nine statistic is well suited to alert policymakers and the general public to the social significance of breast cancer, for example, in an attempt to direct public funding and attention toward breast cancer research, prevention, and treatment. However, the figure is much less appropriate to communicate individual chances of breast cancer to women. Health communicators need to be aware of those differences in context and relevance.

The complexity and challenge of communicating probabilities are certainly not limited to breast cancer and are, perhaps somewhat surprisingly, related not only to patients. A systematic review of the literature on the role of primary care in genetic services reports, "GPs [general practitioners] accept that they have an increasing role to play in genetics, but lack confidence in their ability to do so because of limited knowledge of clinical genetics" (Emery, Watson, Rose, & Andermann, 1999, p. 426). In particular, physicians have been found to interpret proportions incorrectly to a startling degree (Emery et al., 1999).

Gigerenzer and Edwards (2003) argued, "Statistical innumeracy is often attributed to problems inside our minds. We disagree: the problem is not simply internal but lies in the external representation of information, and hence a solution exists. Every piece of statistical information needs a representation—that is, a form. Some forms tend to cloud minds, while others foster insight. We know of no medical institution that teaches the power of statistical representations; even worse, writers of information brochures for the public seem to prefer confusing representations" (p. 741).

We have shown that both patients and health care providers can misinterpret probabilities provided by genetic screenings. Even when understanding probability, many will contrast that scientific information with personal experience. However, statistics are about samples and populations, not individual experience. Physicians face this dilemma daily as they weigh reports in the scientific literature against their own clinical experience, just as patients weigh their prognosis against their and their family's and friend's experiences.

The potential for misunderstanding proportions is compounded by the complex nature of health care decisions, as reflected in our multiple domain model of health literacy. For example, imagine a couple receiving the results of a genetic test informing them of a 10 percent chance that their future children will have a cleft lip. Using examples such as rolling dice, genetic counselors try to explain what a 10 percent chance means. They explain, for example, that it does not mean that one out of every 10 children the couple have will have a cleft lip. The counselors feel that they have given the couple a good understanding of the scientific aspects of this genetic test and what it means. In fact, the couple did understand and have developed a fairly high level of scientific literacy in regard to health.

However, in making a decision to end their pregnancy, stunning the doctors and counselors, the couple considered their own and their first child's experiences because that child does have a cleft lip. They considered the culturally grounded reception the child would likely receive (cultural literacy) and considered their medical insurance situation and their ability to have cosmetic surgery performed (civic literacy). In the end, it was not the scientific literacy that counselors had worked so hard to develop in the couple that made the decision. Scientific literacy may have prompted the decision, but the decision hinged on the other domains of health literacy. Individuals will tend to give weight to the dimensions of health literacy that seem most relevant to them in their daily experiences, often counter to the thinking of medical practitioners who specialize in the scientific domain of health literacy.

Wrapping Up

The sheer complexity of the structure and function of DNA is challenging enough in the best of contexts. A trip to a clinical setting is usually prompted by a health problem and accompanied by higher-than-normal stress levels. That combination taxes a person's health literacy and communication skills and increases the challenge to a successful understanding of medical science as well as the complex metaphors and probabilities often used to communicate about genomics. In turn, this makes informed decision making a difficult goal. Medical practitioners need to reach out through those barriers and communicate simply, efficiently, and effectively. To reach that end, they need training that is too often unavailable.

Successful communication of the biomedical knowledge about health and disease is one of the primary roles of health care providers. Integrally related to that role is a need to establish trust. A broad understanding of the role of health literacy will support doctors, nurses, public health officials, and the entire gamut of health care providers as they build and maintain productive relationships based on shared understanding and trust. If health care providers are aware of each of the domains of health literacy and the role they play in patients' decision-making processes, they will be better prepared to assist their patients.

Exercises

1. Analyze one example of media coverage of genomics using the four domains of health literacy presented in this book.

2. Create a genomics glossary for your own use, and then create one for patients' use. Why are they different?

3. Find as many ways as you can of explaining what a 25 percent chance of a person's future child being born with a certain genetic trait means to them. Which are most successful to you? Ask others as well. Does everyone agree on the best way to communicate probabilities? If not, why not?

10

Highlighting the Role of Civic Literacy
The Massachusetts Tobacco Control Program

Our health literacy evolves and changes through the course of a lifetime. Some of those changes are the result of individual learning, others can develop from new scientific discoveries, and others are the outcomes of shifting social norms or campaigns by governmental and nongovernmental organizations.

In this case study, we highlight how health literacy skills in the domain of civic literacy can promote civic participation, explain the ties between individual and public health, and improve analysis and understanding of mass media content. To do so, we draw on examples from the Tobacco Control Program of the Massachusetts Department of Health. That effort, which continues at much reduced funding levels, was a comprehensive statewide coordinated campaign with elements specifically targeting the civic domain of health literacy.

Smoking and Health: The Threat

About 15 billion cigarettes are smoked each day around the world (Mackay & Eriksen, 2002). In the United States alone, nearly 500,000 people die each year of a tobacco-related illness, making

---

This chapter was prepared with the assistance of Sarah Atunah-Jay.

the use of tobacco the leading preventable cause of premature death in the United States. More people die from tobacco-related causes in the United States than die from homicides, suicides, AIDS, motor vehicle accidents, illegal drugs, and alcohol combined (Centers for Disease Control and Prevention, 2003).

Secondhand smoke, less commonly called environmental tobacco smoke, underlies nearly 3,000 deaths from lung disease and as many as 35,000 deaths from ischemic heart disease among adult nonsmokers each year in the United States. Secondhand smoke pollutes every stage of life, affecting fetal development and causing respiratory disease, cancer, and cardiovascular disease (National Cancer Institute, 1999).

Still, millions of people begin smoking each year despite the risks to themselves and to others. Current trends in smoking indicate that over 5 million people currently under the age of 18 will eventually die from a disease attributable to smoking (Centers for Disease Control and Prevention, 1998b).

Recognizing Secondhand Smoke

In 1986, the U.S. Surgeon General's office published its first report identifying secondhand smoke as a health hazard to nonsmokers (U.S. Department of Health and Human Services, 1986).

Prior to the surgeon general's report, to smoke or not to smoke was generally viewed as a personal choice, mainly causing personal injury. Complaints of smelly hair and clothes did not hold enough weight to move the country to limit smoking in public places. Once secondhand smoke was recognized as a danger to public health, nonsmokers' rights movements began to blossom, and smoking regulations sprang up in schools, government buildings, and the transportation industry (Libby, 1995).

Smoking and Health Literacy

Researchers investigating trends in smoking find that education level, often used as a surrogate measure for fundamental literacy, is closely linked with smoking. Nearly half (47.2 percent) of adults who have earned a general educational development diploma are smokers, while those with master's, professional, and doctoral degrees are the least likely to smoke (8.4 percent) (Centers for Disease Control and Prevention, 2002b). College graduates are the most likely to quit smoking (66.6 percent) and the most likely never to have smoked (66.5 percent), while blue-collar and service workers are the most likely to smoke and are the slowest at quitting (Giovino, 2002).

That relationship between education and smoking, however, does not fully explain why people smoke, as exhibited by the large number of health care providers who smoke. If health literacy were as simple as the possession of medical knowledge about the causes of poor health, smoking would be much easier to eradicate. No matter how easy it is for nonsmokers to presume smokers are simply in denial about the health risks of smoking, such is not the entire case. The difficulty people have stopping smoking, the fact that people continue to start smoking for the first time, and the continued exposure of nonsmokers to secondhand smoke alert us that factors beyond knowledge are at work.

In this chapter, we explore efforts in Massachusetts to reduce the number of smokers and the exposure of nonsmokers to secondhand smoke. This case study demonstrates the role civic literacy plays in healthy choices. However, it is important to keep in mind that there are strong interrelationships among the domains, and no single domain of health literacy operates in a vacuum.

Massachusetts Tobacco Control Program

Fostered by new findings that secondhand smoke is dangerous, Massachusetts passed a law in 1987 that restricted smoking in public places. Later that year, the Massachusetts Department of Public

---

Civic Literacy

Civic literacy is the domain of health literacy related to the abilities that enable citizens to become aware of public issues and involved in the decision-making process. Categories in this domain of health literacy include

- Media literacy skills
- Knowledge of civic and governmental processes
- Awareness that individual health decisions can impact public health

---

Health organized a planning committee of antismoking advocates, health professionals, and voluntary organizations. That committee developed three action areas for the state's tobacco control program (Abt Associates, 2000; Robbins, 2002) that have since been expanded into four main goals for the program:

- Preventing initiation of tobacco use among youth
- Eliminating exposure to environmental tobacco smoke
- Promoting smoking cessation among young people and adults
- Identifying and eliminating tobacco-related disparities in specific population groups

In 1992, Massachusetts voters approved an initiative that increased the tax on tobacco to fund tobacco control efforts (Koh, 2002). The funds created the Massachusetts Tobacco Control Program (MTCP) in October 1993 (Robbins, 2002). In 1999, the program received additional funding from the Centers for Disease Control and Prevention (CDC), and the 1998 national tobacco settlement brought between $13 million and $22 million annually. Thus, the MTCP was very funded for several years, from a high of $52 million in 1993–1994, down to $31 million in 1999. At the time, Massachusetts was first in the nation for funding tobacco prevention and control (Campaign for Tobacco-Free Kids, American Lung Association, American Cancer Association, American Heart Association, & SmokeLess States National Tobacco Policy Initiative, 2003).

Tobacco Master Settlement, 1998

In 1998, the Tobacco Master Settlement Agreement required the tobacco industry to begin paying the 46 participating states in perpetuity, with the amount totaling $206 billion by 2025, to recover costs associated with treating smoking-related illnesses (National Association of Attorney Generals, n.d.). The agreement included strong, but not binding, language indicating that the states were expected to spend between 20 and 25 percent of the money to prevent and reduce tobacco use. The majority of states did not spend the recommended amount on tobacco prevention and control (Campaign for Tobacco-Free Kids, 2003).

In 2003, only 4 states funded tobacco prevention and cessation programs at the minimum levels recommended by the CDC, and only 19 states committed even 50 percent of the minimum recommended funding. That same year, 3 states and the District of Columbia spent none of their settlement money on tobacco prevention (Campaign for Tobacco-Free Kids, 2003).

The MTCP, as a comprehensive campaign, included a mass media campaign, locally organized community programs, and statewide programs designed to support community efforts or deliver services directly to the general population (Abt Associates, 2000). The different aspects of the program were phased in over time, with the media campaign beginning first. The complementary initiatives—mass media, locally organized community-based efforts, and statewide centrally organized support services—made a significant impact on the use and perception of tobacco in Massachusetts.

In Massachusetts, the tobacco control program was indisputably effective. Between 1990 and 1999, the decline in smoking rates among Massachusetts residents surpassed those of states without tobacco control programs. Per capita cigarette consumption dropped by 36 percent, while in other states, consumption dropped by only 16 percent on average (excluding California, which had a comparable program). Smoking by pregnant women dropped from 25 percent to 11 percent, the greatest percentage decline in any state, and smoking among youth dropped 6 percent (from 36 percent to 30 percent) while remaining almost unchanged in the rest of the country (Abt Associates, 2000).

The Mass Media Campaign: Improving Health Literacy

MTCP contracted with an advertising agency, Arnold Communications, to conduct the statewide mass media campaign, which included hundreds of television, radio, newspaper, and billboard advertisements. Mass media efforts were coordinated with community-based efforts throughout the state. Messages focused on preventing youth from starting to smoke, getting current smokers to quit, and reducing exposure to secondhand smoke. The mass media campaign, in particular television and radio, was recognized as an important outlet to reach individuals with lower levels of education, a group that tends to receive higher levels of exposure to secondhand smoke (Abt Associates, 2000).

Both qualitative focus groups and quantitative research helped shape the campaign. For example, a study of focus groups conducted by the California, Massachusetts, and Michigan's antismoking campaigns found that advertisements focusing on tobacco industry manipulation and secondhand smoke were the most effective strate-

---

A Magic Bullet?

According to Jim Hyde, associate professor of family medicine and community health at Tufts University and chair of the Massachusetts Question 1 Tobacco Tax Advisory Committee, finally having sufficient resources to purchase media time and produce first-rate ads, generated an initial enthusiasm and hope that the media campaign could be a silver bullet. (Massachusetts allows referendums to be placed on election ballots. Question 1, which was approved, increased the tax on tobacco products to fund tobacco education and prevention programs.) Belief in a direct and strong media effect—a magic bullet theory—is not uncommon, but there is little empirical evidence to support that notion.

The campaigners soon discovered that "it turned out that was a lunatic notion. Media is not sufficient to change behavior. . . . What really brought the change was the stuff that was happening on the ground at the local level. The media campaign gave visibility to the overall tobacco control effort."

---

gies for "denormalizing" smoking and reducing cigarette consumption (Goldman & Glantz, 1998). Another study, based on a random digit dial telephone survey conducted at the start of the MTCP media campaign and repeated three years later, found that advertisements depicting suffering as a result of tobacco use were effective in promoting quitting and reinforcing the decision to quit (Biener, McCallum-Keeler, & Nyman, 2000).

Targeting Secondhand Smoke

In exploring the role of the civic domain of health literacy, we will look at two specific examples of the MTCP mass media campaign: a television spot named "Baby Monitor" and a banner placed on the sides of public buses.

The dominant visual element during the television commercial is a baby monitor emitting the sound of a baby crying. The commercial is designed to pull directly at the viewers' heartstrings, as young children are held precious in the civic conscious, deserving of special care and protection as they are defenseless.

The text on screen in the commercial begins, "Every year, 300,000 babies get sick from secondhand smoke" (Exhibit 10.1). Action breaks the frame as a shadow of a hand, with suit cuffs

Exhibit 10.1. "Baby Monitor" Television Spot.

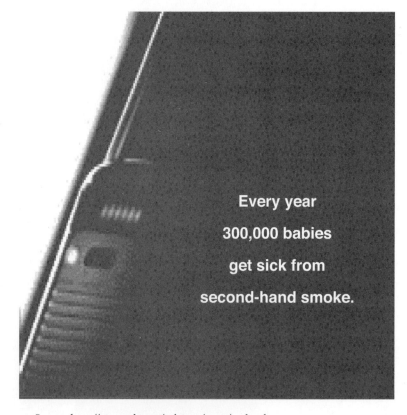

Source: http://www.cdc.gov/tobacco/mcrc/nofees.htm.

implying the individual is a man of business, reaches into the screen to switch off the baby monitor. The cries are cut off. The text now reads, "But the tobacco industry doesn't want to hear it."

In identifying what will be taken as a public and serious issue (babies without means to protect themselves from secondhand smoke) and a source of the problem (the tobacco industry), this TV spot carefully avoids placing blame on parents or individual smokers, the target audiences. Instead, the tobacco industry is effectively framed as an external evildoer everyone should combat in order to save the defenseless child. The spot is an example of civic literacy in action.

Hyde said that the spot "was trying to decouple this issue from people so that we wouldn't be accused of beating up on the poor smoker. It was very powerful and got a lot of attention. It looked so simple but it was incredibly complex and carefully thought through."

In essence, the advertisement informs viewers that an individual's decision to smoke is influenced by other forces and that the decision, once made, can harm the health and well-being of nonsmokers. Those important pieces of information directly increase civic health literacy and can help empower individuals to quit smoking and support antitobacco efforts in their community. In addition, based on research indicating that Spanish- and Portuguese-speaking smokers considered potential harm to children an important motivator to stop smoking, this commercial was translated into both languages.

A sign placed on the side of buses was another element of the Massachusetts campaign (Exhibit 10.2). The poster, brilliant in its simplicity, explicitly links otherwise unconnected individuals to make the connection between secondhand smoke and lung cancer patently clear. The use of buses as a platform for communication reaches a wide audience, not only those who use mass transportation but also those who see the buses pass by.

Exhibit 10.2. Antismoking Banner for Public Buses.

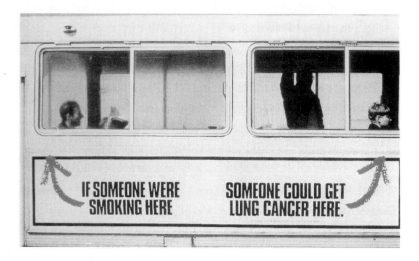

IF SOMEONE WERE
SMOKING HERE

SOMEONE COULD GET
LUNG CANCER HERE.

Civic Action: Mobilizing the Greater Lawrence Community

Another important component of the MTCP allowed individual cities and towns to apply for grants to conduct locally organized tobacco control programs. Local efforts had the freedom to directly tie into the umbrella of the mass media campaign, organize an activity in parallel with the statewide mass media campaign, or plan their own approach.

In 2001, the Greater Lawrence Tobacco Free Community Mobilization Network and the Northeast Tobacco Free Network (http://www.tobaccofreenetwork.org/) joined efforts to organize and enact local regulations to make restaurant dining areas smoke free or make all restaurants and bars 100 percent smoke free.

The effort was based on research into the views of area citizens. For example, "a survey of Methuen registered voters in 2000 found that 60 percent preferred 100 percent smoke-free regulation, 80 percent requested nonsmoking seating and 90 percent would eat out more or the same if Methuen restaurants were smoke-free," reported

Diane Knight, coordinator of the Northeast Tobacco Free Network. However, debates in the local newspaper and comments made at public hearings indicated that some community members remained concerned that smoke-free regulations would deal a major economic blow to restaurants. Thus, individuals needed not only to assess their own feelings on the issue but also to consider community implications.

Aware that smoke-free policies had resulted in no negative economic impacts in other communities, the coalition initiated a print-based testimonial campaign with the ultimate goal of increasing support for smoke-free legislation. Kristen Hill, network coordinator of the Greater Lawrence Tobacco Free Network, explained the communication strategy: "It was a positive strategy focusing on what good was already happening. It educated people to look for smoke-free restaurants; to be aware of smoke-free legislation; raised awareness that smoking is dangerous even in a restaurant; gave a business perspective, spoke from experience; and provided a Web site for more information."

By demonstrating support for the regulations from restaurants and patrons, the advertisement undercut the notion that going smoke free would be bad for business. "The industry was trying to paint that picture," said Jim Ryan, director of the Greater Lawrence Tobacco Free Community Mobilization Network. "We tried to avoid focusing on the negatives of smoking in restaurants. For example, we did not want testimonials such as, 'When someone lights up in a restaurant, I just want to leave.' By focusing on the positive, we hoped to avoid any backlash from smokers and dining establishments that cater to them."

Two of the three communities targeted in the campaign did enact smoke-free regulations, one regulating smoking in bars as well. Although subsequent amendments weakened the initial regulations, the policies are more comprehensive than those before the campaign. Here too, the central message of the campaign focused on elements of the civic domain of health literacy: making connections between individual and public health and the ability to access, understand, and judge between different perspectives in the mass media.

Calls for Action: Youth Participation

Increasing the participation of youth was another component of the MTCP campaign. As a basic approach, youth groups gathered and studied their peers' knowledge, attitudes, and behaviors toward tobacco in order to inform their own strategy development. Their strategy shifted from a peer counseling model to a social action model as health literacy skills transferred the student's newly acquired information to behaviors. As a result, teenagers became effective in influencing local policy changes and in monitoring local tobacco sales to minors, according to Gregory Connolly, director of the Massachusetts Tobacco Control Program.

Teens Against Tobacco, a group based in the Dorchester neighborhood of Boston, succeeded in pressuring the *Boston Globe* to stop printing tobacco ads, established "no-smoking in homes" agreements with local families, and raised awareness of the dangers of tobacco smoke through workshops and health fairs.

"Teens got involved when a couple of nursing students discovered how many people were getting sick from tobacco use in our area," according to Bill Loesch, founder of Teens Against Tobacco. "They worked with a few teens to look at the way stores were advertising in their store windows and glass doors. They taught each other and inspired each other to take on the tobacco giants and industry." (In order to protect the privacy of the minors involved in the program, we are supplying them with fictitious first names.)

The teen groups were fundamentally under the control of the teens themselves, with individuals like Loesch serving as mentors and guides. Donna-Lee, a three-year member of the program, explained, "We have to choose our projects, choose the strategies we're going to take to fulfill that project. . . . We try to educate our peers, people within our same age group. So that's how it's really helpful. Teens, they respond better if it's someone around their age speaking to them."

The teens also found motivation from their own lives. Brandon said, "My father, he was a smoker; I thought if I joined here, I would learn something about tobacco and how it was sick to smoke cigarettes and what the stuff does to you. And I could bring the information home and let him know." The program also helped Ava learn about her own health problems caused by secondhand smoke. She told us, "My mom smokes and so does my aunt, and those are the people that I'm around the most. I knew I had asthma because of secondhand smoke. I'm one of those kids that's always sick. I wanted to see if there's anything that may have been caused by the smoke. When I started researching tobacco, I found that you're at higher risk for ulcers when you have secondhand smoke, and I have an ulcer. You're at higher risk for pneumonia, and my dad died of pneumonia."

She continued, "When I saw those stupid ads [by the tobacco industry] that had cartoons on them, I was like, that's not the reality of cigarettes." Ava witnessed the effects of cigarette smoking on her mother firsthand: "She wasn't happy. Especially the withdrawal periods, those were the worst. When she'd try to quit and she'd be all mean to me and irritated. She'd be up all night and pacing, and I could hear her. I knew that those people on the ads were supposed to be representing my mom, but they're not my mom. Apparently [according to the ads] smoking doesn't do anything to you and you can go to the beach and look great and blah, blah, blah."

Armed with the strength of the group and with their own self-awareness they had created—civic skills—the group set out to educate themselves, their peers, and their communities about the health risks associated with tobacco use. They visited health centers and hospitals to gather more information about tobacco. They applied the information and skills they learned to their community work. One of their first efforts was to establish "Healthy Home and Family" contracts. "It's basically a contract between me and the adult saying that they won't smoke in their home when their kids are present because of secondhand smoke and how deadly it is," said Cynthia about the contracts. "We checked up on the people to make sure they were abiding by the contract. That was just one step to making our communities safer."

Another early, and very public, success for the group occurred when they convinced the *Boston Globe,* the eighth largest-circulation newspaper in the United States, to stop printing tobacco ads. "At that time there were maybe only four of us. A little group. We looked inside the *Globe* and noticed they had these color advertisements for Parliament cigarettes. And if we're looking in the *Globe,* then we know that our peers are looking in the *Globe,* and it attracted our attention, and we were outraged. We were, like, this should not be here," Cynthia said.

After writing letters to the editor and publisher, the teens felt they were being brushed off. They requested and received a meeting. Cynthia remembers, "Their headquarters are right on Morrissey Boulevard, really nice and close. So we're all excited about this meeting. We incorporated a whole bunch of teens in the community who shared our interest in getting the *Globe* to stop advertising and we all went down. But they had us meet with their PR [public relations] guy rather than anybody important. Once again he brushed us off."

That further motivated the teens, and they began a petition drive, obtaining over 2,000 signatures while informing and educating the community in the process. Some thought that the teens could not change the practices of a large corporation. Cynthia said:

> A lot of people discouraged us, saying you guys are just a bunch of kids trying to get this large corporation to stop advertising; it's never going to happen.
>
> We then decided to hold a press conference right in front of the health center telling the community that we have all of these supporters and we want to expose that

the *Globe* does not care that this community doesn't want them to advertise tobacco products. So we informed all the media of this press conference that was going to happen, and the *Globe* was also informed. The day before our press conference they pulled all of their [cigarette] advertisements. They did not want the negative press. They did not want to seem like they didn't care about the community. So then our press conference went about congratulating the *Globe* on not advertising and praising them. . . . They stopped advertising.

The program achieved a great success by increasing the health literacy of the teens and, through them, the community at large. For instance, the teens increased elements of their civic health literacy in regard to health and tobacco use by learning to:

- Judge sources of information about health

- Judge the quality and veracity of information in advertisements

- Understand how marketing efforts can sway decisions

- Access and use a variety of information sources beyond books and the internet

- Gather knowledge and apply it in civic advocacy through letter-writing and petition drives and meeting with officials

Increasing those elements of their civic literacy in regard to their health and the health risks posed by tobacco use, the teen group was able to better protect their own health and their families' health, and to extend that protection to their community and the rest of the state.

Wrapping Up

In 2003, budget cuts all but eliminated the MTCP. Funding was reduced by 90 percent from $48 million to $4.8 million. Nevertheless, some of the state's cities and towns continue to work to pass antismoking regulations, indicating commitment to a cause that really did take root in Massachusetts.

The MTCP is far from alone in terms of successful efforts to address health literacy problems that have seen their budgets cut. A classic example comes from the state of Andra Pradesh in India. A literacy program was established in a way that allowed the female participants to select the content, and the women selected alcohol use, a serious issue in their lives. As a result, the literacy program coalesced into a civic effort that successfully banned alcohol sales. The state, realizing the loss of income from tax on alcohol, eliminated the literacy program and eventually allowed alcohol to be sold again (Mukherjee & Vasanta, 2002).

The clear implication, one that is repeated over years and across continents, is that while improving literacy can pay for itself by reducing the social costs associated with low literacy and poor health, it is important that policymakers are made aware of the true cost reductions associated with improved literacy. Improving the health literacy of everyone, including governmental leaders and decision makers, will produce better outcomes for everyone.

Exercises

1. If you know anyone who smokes, ask this person to explain to you why he smokes. Analyze the response to determine which domains of health literacy are and are not involved in his response.

2. In 1971, the U.S. government banned cigarette advertising on television. The government of India did the same in 2005.

Find a source of data on smoking rates, and determine if the advertising bans have had any effect.

3. A well-known series of advertisements by Camel cigarettes featured the cartoon character Joe Cool. Find examples of Joe Cool on the internet, and determine what audience the advertising campaign was targeted. Using the domains of health literacy, explain how Joe Cool was effective.

4. In this book, we argue that health literacy is multidimensional and an effective way to enhance individuals' ability to act in their and others' best interest. Discuss the implications of that for each of the following:

Elected officials

Unelected policymakers

Physicians

Insurance companies

Journalists

11

Highlighting the Role
of Cultural Literacy, Part 1
The Changing Face of HIV/AIDS

Sub-Saharan Africa, Ryan White, Rock Hudson, white-cloaked medical researchers, Magic Johnson, a gay disease, UNAIDS, condoms, the WHO's 3 × 5 initiative, and red ribbons are among the many public faces of acquired immune deficiency syndrome, or AIDS, and human immunodeficiency virus, HIV.

Initially, it was thought of as a disease confined to homosexuals, heroin users, Haitians, and the homeless, but it is clear that HIV/AIDS does not discriminate. Infection is not dependent on identity. Public awareness campaigns, galvanized by the urgency of the epidemic and the panic that it engendered, originally aimed to uniformly distribute knowledge about the disease and prevention. However, over the past two decades, messages and campaigns have evolved into coordinated and targeted efforts reflecting the increasing scientific understandings of HIV/AIDS and the process of encouraging behavior change. These changes provide important and intriguing lessons about the role of the cultural domain of health literacy.

The culture and science of medicine defines AIDS as a disease resulting from a viral infection, HIV, and has identified vectors of transmission, such as unprotected sex, sharing needles, and tainted

---

This chapter was prepared with the assistance of Shusmita Dhar.

blood supplies. The many cultures of the United States and the rest of the world, however, have different and changing understandings of HIV/AIDS. In the early 1980s, the strongest belief in the United States was that AIDS was a disease limited to the homosexual community. Some people with strong conservative religious beliefs continue to believe that AIDS is God's retribution for a "sinful" life, and some conspiracy theorists persist in the belief that AIDS is the result of a government-run biomedical experiment gone awry.

While those misperceptions may represent extremes, their persistence indicates some of the cultural barriers to effective health communication and care. Such barriers are not solely a public problem, as cultural perceptions of HIV/AIDS influence the progress of biomedical research and the provision of health care. Efforts to reduce and stop the spread of HIV/AIDS must be designed with cultural literacies in mind.

Cultural Literacy

Cultural literacy, as a domain of health literacy, refers to the abilities to recognize and use collective beliefs, customs, worldview, and social identity in order to interpret and act on health information. This domain includes a recognition and skill on the communicator's part to frame health information to accommodate powerful cultural understandings of health information, science, and individual and collective action

---

Culture is not merely a function of race, nationality, or geography. Culture can be centered in a country but also crosses political boundaries, spans the globe, or resides in a small neighborhood. Cultures can be based on occupation, lifestyle, or origin. Our culturally grounded understandings of the world form the basic outlines within which we operate. Those outlines are not fixed. The ability to influence culture is the ability to influence common sense, or the basic set of conceptions and categories that form the practical consciousness of people (Hall, 1996).

In this chapter, we review the emergence and spread of HIV/AIDS and briefly outline some of the trends and events in the public dialogue about HIV/AIDS in the United States. We focus on selected campaigns and their successes and failures in incorporating elements of cultural literacy.

Culture and Health

Introducing culture into a discussion of health literacy builds on an understanding of health as a culturally dependent concept. There is not a globally valid definition of health, as what it means to be "healthy" changes between individuals, communities, cultures, and across time and context. Expectations of health differ, for example, between an adult with HIV, a teenager, a 92-year-old, a subsistence farmer in Indonesia, a banker in South Africa, or a homeless woman in New York City.

Many studies assessing efforts to introduce culture into HIV/AIDS education and intervention projects often rely primarily on ethnicity and race to define culture (Wilson & Miller, 2003). This is a dangerous oversimplification of culture, producing two equally unfortunate misunderstandings: that whites of predominantly European heritage set the gold standard against which other cultures are judged, and that culture is solely encountered in traditionally marginalized groups.

HIV/AIDS in the United States

In the United States, the first case of what would soon be known as AIDS was reported in 1981. The public response mainly consisted of denial or blame. In February 1982, the Centers for Disease Control and Prevention (CDC) reported that 251 Americans had what was then called gay-related immunodeficiency syndrome. By early 1988, the caseload hit 50,000, doubling to 100,000 in 1989. By 1993, AIDS was the leading cause of death among those 25 to 44 years old, and no one was able to deny the threat of HIV/AIDS (Shilts, 1988; see Figure 11.1).

The public face of HIV/AIDS has changed a great deal since the early 1980s, and the image of HIV/AIDS as a plague among homosexuals, hemophiliacs, the homeless, and Haitians has faded. Yet there is continuing cause for concern. The number of new cases has hovered at just over 40,000 per year since 1998 as the rate of decline has slowed from 13 percent in 1997 to 3 percent in 1999 (Centers for Disease Control, 2001). The story is not the same for all groups. Between 1996 and 1997, incidence among whites dropped roughly 25 percent (from 21,498 to 16,038), whereas among Hispanics, the number of new cases fell by roughly 17 percent (from 11,920 to

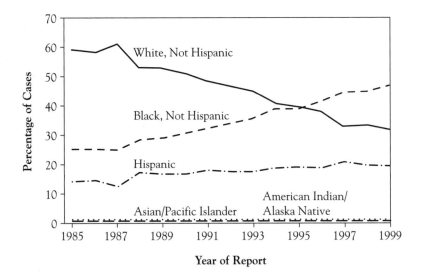

Figure 11.1. Proportion of AIDS Cases in the United States, by Race/Ethnicity and Year of Report, 1985–1999.

Source: Centers for Disease Control (2001).

9,864), and among blacks incidence declined by only around 13 percent (from 26,610 to 23,151).

While blacks represent around 12 percent of the general population in the United States, they experience roughly 54 percent of new infections (Centers for Disease Control, 2001). Women are at increasing risk as well, accounting for 14 percent of all new AIDS cases in 1992 and 20 percent in 1999. In 1997, AIDS became the leading cause of death for women between ages 25 and 44 in New York City. There is also a resurgence of cases in young men who have sex with men, as incidence rose from 15,962 in 2000 to 16,453 a year later (Centers for Disease Control, 2001). The battle against HIV/AIDS is clearly far from won; attitudes toward the disease, behavior patterns of young gay men, and increasing rates of gonorrhea and syphilis suggest that HIV incidence is likely to rise further (Wolitski, Valdiserri, Denning, & Levine, 2001).

The Public Dialogue

Silence defined the initial response to HIV/AIDS (Shilts, 1988). The *New York Times*, so often the agenda setter for American mass media, did not publish a front-page article on HIV/AIDS until 1983 (Singhal & Rogers, 2003). President Ronald Reagan did not give a speech on the topic until 1987 (Singhal & Rogers, 2003).

HIV/AIDS was perhaps most notably brought to the public agenda through the work of Randy Shilts in the *San Francisco Chronicle*, but also in alternative newspapers and magazines across the country and through the work of activist organizations and public health departments. Slowly, denial of the threat of AIDS became an untenable position.

The list of famous figures and events having an impact on the public dialogue and opinion about HIV/AIDS is unfortunately incomplete but already includes Rock Hudson, 13-year-old hemophiliac Ryan White, Ronald Reagan's apology for neglecting the epidemic, three-time NBA Most Valuable Player Earvin "Magic"

Johnson, tennis great Arthur Ashe, Olympic figure skater John Curry, Randy Shilts, and Olympic medalist Greg Louganis.

Such public events have influenced public opinion. For example, Magic Johnson's announcement of his HIV-positive status and use of his celebrity status to increase awareness of HIV/AIDS is argued to have increased the level of accurate knowledge, the number of individuals being tested for HIV, the level of interest in obtaining information about HIV/AIDS, and the perception of vulnerability to HIV/AIDS in the general population (Casey et al., 2003).

Overall, there has been a general increase in the correct information held by Americans about the means of infection of HIV/AIDs and a decrease in the misinformation about how HIV/AIDS can be transmitted. Nevertheless, HIV/AIDS is still misunderstood by many. In 2000, a national poll found that 10 percent of respondents believed people could get HIV/AIDS from a toilet seat; 15 percent believed it was possible to get from sharing glasses, silverware, or plates; and 31 percent of the respondents believed people could get HIV/AIDS by kissing (Aragon, Kates, Greene, & Hoff, 2001).

The Conflict in Communicating About HIV/AIDS

HIV/AIDS was a disease with no effective treatment for some time and is still without a cure. As a result, prevention and testing must be the primary focus of public health efforts. In order to communicate lessons about prevention, culturally sensitive issues must be addressed. In a country where sex education is often couched in euphemisms like "the birds and the bees" or packaged solely as the promotion of sexual abstinence, messages about sex, homosexuality, and drug use that the people need to hear often conflict with cultural norms.

The abstract and unemotional language of science and a reliance on top-down, expert-driven approaches to communication is often the first refuge for a health communicator worried about the potential for cultural-based misunderstandings and backlash. Cultural awareness, sometimes referred to as cultural competency, is a necessary component of successful communication in such instances. As Singhal and Rogers (2003) argue, "Prevention programs need to be non-judgmental, to avoid stigmatizing the particular lifestyles or other behaviors of individuals targeted for prevention activities" (p. 54).

The U.S. Government Acts: "America Responds to AIDS"

In 1987, the CDC launched a multimillion-dollar public education campaign about AIDS, "America Responds to AIDS."

The advertising agency Ogilvy and Mather designed the campaign's centerpiece, an eight-page brochure, "Understanding AIDS," that, in a move matched only by the postcard during the anthrax threat (see Chapter 9), was sent to every household in the country during May and June 1988. The brochure's main focus, in an attempt to correct misunderstandings about AIDS, was on risky behaviors and how people can and cannot get AIDS (Woods, 1991).

Reflecting the central purpose of the brochure to counter misinformation, the language is objective and somewhat removed, lacking the elements of content and style that could create personal relevance for at-risk individuals. For example, repeated references to vaginal or oral sex go without explanation. While many may understand those terms, researchers have demonstrated that individuals living in high-risk cities who found those terms difficult were more likely to report that they had not had vaginal or anal intercourse with others (Binson & Catania, 1998). The direct implication is that sexual activity may be underreported by individuals who should be likely candidates for education and intervention efforts.

Furthermore, while the target audience for the campaign was every American, culturally biased messages are present throughout. The majority of the pictures are of white individuals, and the majority of the discourse accepts the assumption that AIDS is mainly a gay disease. The seeds for victim blaming based on cultural stereotypes were sown throughout this publication. For example, in an inside section, the phrase, "No matter what you may have heard, AIDS is hard to get and is easily avoided," encourages readers to believe that people had to work hard to acquire AIDS and that choices related to sexual preference are easy to change. Misinformation about AIDS transmission and negative attitudes toward homosexuals are strong predictors of support for stringent restrictions of persons with AIDS (Price & Hsu, 1992).

Effects of the campaign were, frankly, minimal. A Gallup Poll on July 20, 1988, found that 63 percent of the respondents who remembered receiving the brochure, 82 percent of those reporting reading the brochure, and 51 percent of those reporting receiving the brochure said they had discussed it with others. Unfortunately, a majority (65 percent) said the brochure added little or nothing to their knowledge about AIDS. In perhaps the greatest, yet counterproductive, effect potentially attributable to the campaign, there was roughly a 20 percent increase in the number of people expressing concern about AIDS as an epidemic everyone faced. In addition to that general increase in fear of AIDS, the campaign may also have played a role in increasing fears about contracting AIDS while giving blood (Singer, Rogers, & Glassman, 1988).

At the time, many educational efforts from the public health sector carried those sorts of messages. There was little in the way of practical advice, preventive messages, or behavior interventions. A typical campaign in this mode, by the public health department of San Francisco, featured the slogan "Fight the Fear with Facts" (see Exhibit 11.1.). These advertisements feature a series of inanimate objects as the dominant visual element: doorknobs, a bus seat, hot tub, or water fountains. Underneath the image were the words, "Some people think you can catch AIDS from [the featured object]." While the information presented in this campaign was correct and needed, it was not put into a context relevant to many readers. The

Exhibit 11.1. A Fact-Filled, Nontargeted
Advertisement for AIDS Education.

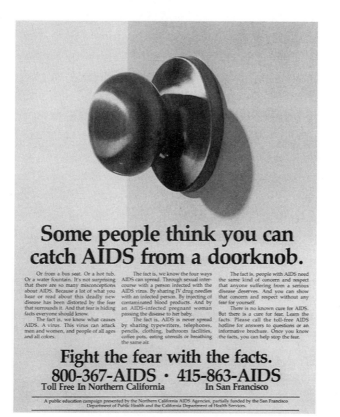

priority of this campaign was clearly to transfer information, not
bring about behavior change, so at best, the ads prevented the infor-
mational climate about AIDS from further deterioration.

In general, the initial, large-scale public campaigns addressing
the emergence of HIV/AIDS, such as the CDC's "America Responds
to AIDS," shared a broad assumption that simply providing correct
information would lead to prevention and that information alone
could defeat cultural stereotypes about homosexuals and AIDS.

Early Responses at the Community Level

Community-based organizations in major metropolitan areas, rather than government agencies, created the initial efforts directly targeting behavior change. As early as 1982, the San Francisco AIDS Foundation and the Gay Men's Health Crisis in New York City were undertaking prevention education as a central mission.

Armed with ambition, a sense of urgency, and an intrinsic understanding of their constituencies, community-based organizations in urban areas designed and orchestrated targeted awareness and prevention campaigns. Many of these groups were formed by groups of gay men motivated and moved to action by a disease that they saw as disproportionately affecting their community. They had a sense of how to speak about sex and behavior, what kind of language would be meaningful and effective, and what images and messages would be culturally relevant within their communities.

For example, the STOP AIDS (http://www.stopaids.org) movement in San Francisco showed that these kinds of messages could be successful (Singhal & Rogers, 2003). Relying on peer educators, often who were HIV positive themselves, to design and implement prevention messages, the resulting campaigns were targeted at the large and relatively open gay community in the city. From 1983 to 1987, self-reports of nonmonogamous men having unprotected anal intercourse fell from 71 percent to 21 percent (Singhal & Rogers, 2003). Two reasons for this success are that the campaign "(a) was highly targeted to a specific population of high risk individuals; (b) was founded and implemented by respected leaders of the target community rather than by 'outside' professionals, organizers, or educators" (Singhal & Rogers, 2003, p. 168).

Early examples of targeted campaigns that worked shaped the future of HIV/AIDS prevention education in the United States. They used direct, clear, and relevant language to describe sex and couched a call for individual action within the context of a greater community.

From Minimizing Fear to Changing Behavior:
The National Strategy Shifts

One of the key lessons learned from HIV/AIDS prevention and education efforts is that in order to be effective, communication has to be culturally appropriate for the target audience.

Early responses to AIDS are perhaps best characterized by the San Francisco AIDS Foundation's description of itself: "An emergency response to an emergency health crisis." However, learning from experience, the CDC began to directly fund the prevention efforts of community-based organizations in 1989 (Valdiserri, 2003). The reasoning was natural and reinforces our explicit addition of a cultural domain to health literacy: prevention must focus on modifying behavior, yet we all draw on a complex set of beliefs, habits, and experience—culture—in our decisions about health.

Communicating in a Culturally Literate Way

In order to successfully address cultural literacy issues in communicating, the following attributes must be present:

- The information has to be understandable, written in language and with words that are appropriate for the targeted audience.

- The information must be relevant to the target population.

- The information must be in a form and a location that is accessible and natural for the target population.

- The messages cannot be perceived as off-putting, offensive, or judgmental.

- The campaigns must be responsive to a community's concerns and realities.

Early campaigns had difficulties meeting these goals. They often contained too much information that was at too high a reading level, assumed too much of the audience, and neglected differences in cultural understandings and practices. These campaigns helped fuel attacks by gay activists that federal and state agencies were half-hearted or fueled by discrimination against homosexuals (Epstein, 1995, 2000; Shilts, 1988).

In contrast to the early top-down efforts, community-based organizations have several innate advantages in creating culturally appropriate campaigns:

- Knowledge and familiarity with local idioms and patterns of language use

- Ready access to the community

- An understanding of the community's concerns and questions

- A position of trust within the community

- Knowledge of, and an ability to recruit, respected community leaders as "early adopters" to help influence social and cultural norms (Singhal & Rogers, 2003)

While it is often quite challenging to prove causality when speaking about social phenomena, rates of rectal and pharyngeal gonorrhea declined in New York City during a time period that was coincident with a period of heightened awareness fueled by community-based organizations (Bailey, 1991). A report from a nine-city study concludes that HIV education was effective only when it was produced by groups that could make materials that were "appropriate for and responsive to the lifestyle, language, and environment of the members of that population" (Bailey, 1991, p. 702).

CDC Guidelines

The CDC issued its first guidelines highlighting the importance of community-based planning in 1993 with the goal of improving the effectiveness of prevention programs by strengthening the scientific base, community relevance, and focus of prevention interventions. The principal objectives were to:

- Foster the openness and participatory nature of the community planning process

- Ensure that the community planning group reflects the diversity of the epidemic in that area and that relevant expertise is included

- Ensure that priority HIV prevention needs are determined based on an epidemiological profile and needs assessment

- Ensure that explicit consideration is given to priority needs, outcome effectiveness, cost effectiveness, theory, and community norms and values

- Strive to foster strong, logical linkages among the community planning process, plans, applications for federal funding, and allocation of HIV prevention resources

State health departments across the country generally employed this model in making decisions about funding projects. Thus, rather than launching their own top-down prevention projects, departments of health often partnered with local organizations that serve the communities most at risk. In that way, most, if not all, HIV public health education became community based.

Community Planning:
The San Francisco AIDS Foundation

The San Francisco AIDS Foundation (SFAF) is one of the oldest community-based HIV/AIDS organizations. Founded in 1982 in the Castro district of San Francisco, one of the epicenters of the epidemic, the organization's history and current campaigns provide examples of the power of cultural literacy and the ability of community-based organizations to stay in tune with the changing reality of HIV/AIDS.

Motivated individuals, often personally affected by AIDS, founded the organization. They set about creating educational materials that made sense and that they felt would be effective based on their knowledge and intuition about the audience they were trying to reach: their peers. The results were campaigns that were explicit, sometimes controversial, and often arresting.

As the epidemic was reaching beyond the gay white male community in which the organization had its roots, SFAF extended efforts to other affected communities. To meet the need for messages geared toward intravenous drug users, gay men who were also intravenous drug users were charged with planning the organization's campaigns in this direction. The efforts produced billboards with a picture of a large syringe, carrying the words, "Don't share." The message did not condemn drug use and became controversial in the broader community, but it did reflect the perceptions of the creators and the community they were trying to reach.

From these beginnings, SFAF has developed a process of creating prevention and education campaigns that are responsive to immediate and local concerns and needs by involving members of the target audience early and often. SFAF education committees consult detailed, current, epidemiological data in order to determine what populations demonstrate a need. Qualitative interviews and focus groups are then conducted with members of these target populations, including both HIV-positive and -negative individuals. These studies are used to pinpoint issues that are the most important, the most prohibitive barriers, or specific practices or beliefs that may hinder a prevention message. Information about language, social networks, and possible effective messages or images is sought. Graphic designers and project coordinators incorporate this information in drafts of the proposed campaign. Draft campaign materials are then tested in additional focus groups to assess their appropriateness, effectiveness, and impacts.

SFAF also engages in internal and external evaluation of its efforts. Street polling is done to determine saturation level and assess what kinds of meaning the advertisements have had for different segments of the population.

The results are often effective, timely, and specific to a given problem or barrier. For example, in 1993, the revelation that the drug ecstasy was playing a role in young people's risky behavior prompted a campaign of psychedelic posters and postcards placed in public bathrooms and schools. The message was to try to stay safe, be responsible, and take care of oneself when using the drug.

Focus groups were also used to investigate a resurgence of infection in young gay men and revealed a pattern of assumptions that people made about their sexual partners. For instance, people generally assumed that their partner and they had the same status. Positive individuals assumed others were positive, and HIV-negative individuals assumed others were negative. The resulting, "How do you know what you know?" campaign included explicit images of men engaged in sex, each making potentially erroneous assumptions.

In another example of culturally targeting messages, infection rates identified a need for a campaign to target men in the Tenderloin district of San Francisco ("tenderloin" is a term historically used to refer to less-than-favorable sections of a city. Of course, that is a subjective designation. Roughly, this one refers to an area of San Francisco west of Union Square, south of Nob Hill, east of the Van Ness corridor, and north of Market Street). To address this group, a new branch of SFAF, Black Brothers Esteem, was formed. Focus groups revealed that an issue of particular concern is the sex-for-drugs trade. In the exchange of drugs for sex, HIV prevention is often forgotten.

After initial focus groups, campaigns went through multiple revisions, informed by target audience feedback. For example, there was concern that the early versions were overly romanticized but then that the revisions were overly grim. The messages were trimmed and shaped to their final balance as a result of this continuing input from community members. Decisions on where to place the advertisements and what form they would take were also informed by these discussions. The result has been a highly visible, highly culturally literate campaign.

Specific aspects of this campaign are striking and illustrate the role of cultural literacy. For example, the language used is the slang of the Tenderloin district. "Fair Exchange" referred to the fact that sex for drugs may be considered a fair exchange, but adding HIV infection to the transaction is another matter. "Toss or Tossed" was a reference to the power dynamic in homosexual relationships and how prevention of HIV can enter into this dynamic. The images are stark and striking, drawn in an angular realism, with expressive faces and realistic locales and backgrounds. These ads are then placed in key, visible locations such as on buses and the sides of buildings.

The relationship between organizations like SFAF and their communities becomes even more evident when looking at changes in the campaigns. For example, in contrast to the Tenderloin-based effort, SFAF launched an effort in 1993, Street Smarts, that targeted young male prostitutes who were often fleeing abusive homes and ended up on the street. This campaign, however, was geared toward the Polk Gulch area of San Francisco, a very different cultural context from the Tenderloin district. The message, visually and linguistically different from the stark and blunt message of the Black Brothers Esteem ads, is empowering for a younger population. The people depicted in this campaign are young, white, and wearing leather jackets in visuals that do not resonate with a pop-influenced brightly colored realism; rather, they are grainy, gritty photographs.

These examples demonstrate that if neither the medium nor the content of communication is selected with cultural context in mind, a failure of a population to get a particular message is actually a failure of the message and the messenger to engage the population appropriately. By encouraging and supporting the work of community-based organizations, the CDC and state departments of health are increasing the likelihood that campaigns will incorporate cultural literacy skills and increasing the likelihood that the campaigns will have the desired results.

The rhetoric of community participation, however, is not a blind panacea. It raises its own host of questions:

- How narrowly do the groups have to be defined?

- Are there general principles that can be taken for granted across groups? Across time? Across communities and countries?

- If community-based planning has been successfully endorsed and implemented, why are we still seeing the devastating impact of disease on segments of our populations?

- What lessons have the past presented that can be used to sharpen the effects of community planning in the future?

These questions have to be asked, and asked again, in the planning, creation, and implementation of communication campaigns in the effort to improve decision making and promote healthy choices.

Experience has shown that culture is a more complex and finely tuned concept than often thought; it is much more than race and ethnicity. Researchers have found, for instance, that black and His-panic men who have sex with men may not identify themselves as gay but as participating in a one-off sexual act even if it has occurred several times. Those individuals may not relate to ads geared toward gay men. In addition, adolescent girls, female sex workers, and Latina women may all need to hear the same basic prevention mes-sages, but their very different beliefs, environments, language, and sets of priorities are important to how those messages can be most effectively delivered.

Culture as well is not static. This may help to explain the resur-gence of infection rates in young gay men because they are a sig-nificantly different population from the gay men who founded groups like SFAF and Gay Men's Health Alliance (GMHA) in New York City. Recognition of this ongoing dynamic is vitally important in creating effective campaigns.

Wrapping Up

In this chapter, we have shown a transition in approach from broad-based general education campaigns with limited effectiveness to a growing emphasis on culturally literate, targeted communication efforts led by community-based organizations. These latter efforts increase the likelihood of incorporating appropriate cultural ele-ments through direct and early community involvement that in-creases the likelihood of positive effects.

Importantly, health care communicators must remember that when addressing culture, the ultimate goal is not to produce one ad for each imaginable subpopulation, but to produce coordinated and appropriate campaigns that are more effective across the board. Although one cultural perspective does not fit all populations, employing effective cultural literacy practices in the planning, cre-ation, design, and implementation of communication campaigns certainly does.

Exercises

1. Conduct a small-scale survey among your peers, your family and friends, those you live with, or your neighborhood. Ask individuals how HIV/AIDS can and cannot be transmitted, their level of education, their age, gender, racial/ethnic background, views on homosexuality, religious background, political affiliation, and how much time they spend watching television or reading newspapers. Are there are any correlations among those variables? Why, or why not?

2. What was the last large public event you can think of related to HIV/AIDS? Does that event indicate the trend in the epidemiology of the disease? How, or how not?

3. Visit the web sites of the World Health Organization (http://www.who.int) or UNAIDS (http://www.unaids.org) and learn about the trends of HIV/AIDS around the world. Look at what is being done in various countries in attempts to slow the spread of HIV/AIDS. Do you see any similarities between the early years of HIV/AIDS education campaigns in the United States and what is occurring at the global level?

12

Highlighting the Role
of Cultural Literacy, Part 2
Diabetes and Native Americans

Culture is a concept that carries many meanings, implications, and questions. What is culture? How can we identify culture? What does culture have to do with health literacy? Can an understanding of culture help health care professionals in their quest to improve the health status of individuals and the public at large?

In this case study, we take the position that the answer to the last question is unequivocally yes. Unfortunately, the everyday vagaries of the use of the word have led *culture* to be blamed for too much harm as well as credited for too much good. We do not refer to culture in the sense of high and low, cultured or not. Culture may have a lot do with the choice to get dressed up and go to the symphony or opera, but culture is found not only at the symphony. Indeed, culture is in coffee shops, bus stations, shopping malls, and dance studios. Culture is in Bombay as it is in Burbank.

Culture is the sum of the shared characteristics of a group of people, including language, patterns of behavior, beliefs, identity, customs, traditions, and other modes of expression. These learned characteristics enable group members to hold and communicate shared meanings.

On a more practical level, the ability to influence culture is the ability to influence common sense, or the basic set of conceptions

---

This chapter was prepared with the assistance of Sarah Atunah-Jay and Kibbe Conti.

and categories that form the practical consciousness of people (Hall, 1996). Health literacy, in a very straightforward manner, is the measure of an individual's practical ability to make healthy decisions.

How to Be Culturally Relevant

As we discussed in Chapter One, there are two ends to the broad spectrum of approaches to health promotion, education, and communication. At one end is the historically dominant approach, an expert-driven model. Participatory approaches are at the opposite end of the spectrum.

An expert-driven approach (also called a top-down or deficit model) of communicating to patients and the public is generally based on an assumption of a lack of knowledge that must be remedied, as well as an assumption that possession of that knowledge will result in the desired behavior. From the outset, this approach creates a power differential between provider and community. There is no provision for feedback from the community. Culture, ethical values, attitudes, and behaviors are therefore judged from within a narrow context. In the worst cases, culture is not privileged and becomes stereotyped. Examples include the stereotypes that Latino males are macho and Southeast Asian patients are deferential.

Despite a cutting and valid critique, the expert-driven model has been employed in a wide range of personal and public health problems, not without some notable successes. However, the power differential inherent in the expert-driven approach has hindered its effectiveness, particularly as health issues become more complex. Those diminishing returns result from basic conflicts between the expert model and individuals' belief in their own self-efficacy, adherence to personal worldviews and habits, the evolution of culture, competing definitions of what it is to be healthy, changing patterns of health care provision, and the evolving nature of challenges to good health.

Alternatively, a participatory approach focuses on working with community members. In this approach, voices from the community are empowered and encouraged to define and change goals, decide the way a program is conducted, and define success or failure based on their own needs versus what others have determined is needed (Park, 1993; Pleasant et al., 2003; Zarcadoolas, Timm, & Bibeault, 2001). Cultural values and local context are built into the process by being actively included from the outset.

The participatory approach is being adopted with increasing frequency. That shift in strategy impacts every stage of efforts to improve individual and public health from conceptual design to evaluation. The participatory approach redefines exactly who should be considered an expert. As Cargo et al. (2003) argue in their article focusing on a diabetes prevention effort in a Mohawk community, participatory approaches "allow multiple voices to be heard and establish a process for dialogue in the development and implementation of culturally appropriate interventions" (p. 178). Satisfaction with such efforts is generally high among participants. Effectiveness and impact of the participatory approach are beginning to be documented, but there remain challenges.

This case study explores the role of cultural literacy as a domain of health literacy. We accomplish that task by first describing the prevalence and impact of diabetes in Native American communities and then discussing programs seeking to address the epidemic of diabetes among Native American populations in the United States.

Diabetes and Native Americans: An Epidemic of Culture

No stronger evidence than the prevalence, morbidity, and mortality related to diabetes in Native American communities is needed to justify our choice of material for this case highlighting the role of cultural literacy in health literacy.

Diabetes is the seventh leading cause of the death in the United States and affects 6.3 percent of the total population (18.2 million people). The disease disproportionately affects minority populations. Blacks, Latino Americans, American Indians, and Alaska Natives all have a higher prevalence of diabetes than non-Hispanic whites. American Indians and Alaska Natives have the highest prevalence of diabetes (14.9 percent of those over age 20) of any racial/ethnic group studied and are 2.6 times as likely to have diabetes as non-Hispanic whites of a similar age (National Institute of Diabetes and Digestive and Kidney Diseases, 2003). While rates vary, the Pima tribe in southern Arizona has the highest prevalence, at about 50 percent of individuals between the ages of 30 and 64 years old (Gohdes, 1995). Diabetes is becoming increasingly common in Native American youth (National Diabetes Information Clearinghouse, 2002).

American Indians and Alaska Natives are subject to many predictive risk factors for diabetes. On average, they are among the poorest and least educated groups in the United States and have suffered through a long history of social marginalization. Low socioeconomic status is one of the most powerful risk factors for poor health outcomes (Commission on Macroeconomics and Health, 2001). The Diabetes Surveillance System of the Centers for Disease Control and Prevention found that individuals with at least a high school education are more likely to report employing preventive care practices than those without (National Center for Chronic Disease Prevention and Health Promotion, 2001). Many studies have found similar indicators resulting in poor access to medical care (Weller et al., 1999).

Meeting the challenges of diabetes control is not easy. Understanding the complicated disease process may be difficult. Self-monitoring can be invasive, requiring a blood sample, and time-consuming. Further increasing the barriers, preventive measures such as weight control through diet and exercise may conflict with a patient's lifestyle preferences and cultural norms. Finally, if the

What Is Diabetes?

The American Diabetes Association (http://www.diabetes.org) defines diabetes mellitus as a disease in which the body does not produce or properly use insulin. Insulin is a hormone needed to convert sugar, starches, and other food into energy needed for daily life. There are three types of diabetes. Type 1 diabetes occurs when the body fails to produce insulin. Type 2 diabetes, the most common, occurs when the body develops resistance to insulin. Gestational diabetes occurs during pregnancy when a mother develops insulin resistance.

Hypoglycemia (or low blood sugar) and hyperglycemia (or high blood sugar) are two conditions that occur when the body is lacking or unable to properly use insulin. Both conditions can be extremely serious if not treated properly and necessitate awareness of good diabetes control and recognition of accompanying symptoms.

People with diabetes are at high risk for developing serious health problems, including heart disease, strokes, high blood pressure, blindness, kidney disease, nervous system disease, dental disease, and complications of pregnancy. The health complications that can arise in diabetic patients make preventive care essential for maintaining good health. Education, diet, exercise, weight control, medication, blood glucose self-monitoring, and foot care are important to ensure good control of diabetes.

disease cannot be controlled through lifestyle and behavior change, oral or injectable medications are invasive and complicated and require patient self-management and treatment adherence.

In the case of diabetes, the challenges to individuals with low health literacy are high. The lenses of cultural disenfranchisement and racial prejudice serve to magnify the challenges. Thus, the domain of cultural literacy is one that health care professionals must pay particular attention to.

The Role of Culture in Diabetes Prevention and Care

Cultural literacy is an important element of health care and prevention, made all the more critically important by diseases whose prevalence patterns echo cultural boundaries or practices. A few examples of the positive impact of addressing culture in health care include these:

- A study at a pediatric clinic in Boston found that lack of cultural understanding by staff was one of the top reasons that Latino parents did not bring their children in for an appointment (Flores, Abreu, Olivar, & Kastner, 1998).

- Focus groups conducted with tribal leaders, Indian health professionals, and American Indian community members found a strong preference for diabetes education materials that were relevant to a specific tribe or culture (Robideaux et al., 2000).

- Addressing diverse needs of specific ethnic groups and people of various literacy levels through the use of appropriate tools and techniques has resulted in better diabetes care (Gohdes, 1988).

Hugh Baker, director of the Mandan, Hidatsa, and Arikara Nation's Social Services Office on the Fort Berthold Indian reservation in North Dakota, has long experience with Native American health care programs. Baker believes the success of substance abuse programs that took a culturally grounded approach offers an important lesson for diabetes prevention and other health campaigns. He told us:

I've watched the Indian people try to participate in some kind of recovery program regarding [alcohol] addiction for many years, and it's my earlier experience that they continuously failed when using traditional 12-step programs. By traditional, I mean Anglo models. The only thing that made sense to me, or others, was to look at the recovery process as Indians. To look at the traditional parts, the cultural parts, and what it was really doing to us spiritually and otherwise.

Baker believes that a culturally sensitive approach can benefit all programs, not just those aimed at American Indians: "Probably only in the last 10 or 20 years have we really looked at or changed our focus from being worldwide to becoming more community specific. When we changed that and started looking more at how we can change ourselves using our own philosophies and beliefs, it worked."

There is evidence that the more traditional lifestyles of American Indians, Africans, and Hispanics, with diets low in fat and including daily activities such as walking, gardening, farming, and other forms of physical labor, result in low rates of unhealthy weight gain and diabetes. However, weight gain and often diabetes increasingly occur when individuals from these cultural groups adopt a high-fat diet and inactive lifestyle more typical of contemporary lifestyles in high-income nations. Some researchers think that if prevention and care programs were crafted and conducted in a culturally appropriate manner and if these populations returned to a diet and lifestyle reflecting historic patterns, the risk of diabetes would be reduced, and individuals who have the disease would live healthier lives (National Institute of Diabetes and Digestive and Kidney Diseases, n.d.).

Ethics and fairness demand that such a transition in lifestyle for a health gain should not negatively influence the ability to participate and compete in the global society. As characterized by the Ottawa Charter for Health Promotion, health should be considered a resource for living. Thus, an emphasis on empowering individuals should not necessarily mean that risk is privatized so that the entire burden and responsibility for health falls on the individual. From that perspective, people have a right to health.

In practice, the matter is rarely simple. Day-to-day realities, ethical considerations about personal choice, and the fact that culture evolves and changes differently for different individuals make the ideal scenario more of a theory than a proven practice. Despite the host of challenges, however, several programs are taking up the challenge.

The Sioux San Hospital Diabetes Program

The Sioux San Hospital of Rapid City, South Dakota, is an Indian Health Service hospital. The hospital received federal funding to operate a diabetes prevention and treatment clinic in 2001. Two nurses, a physician's assistant, two registered dietitians, and a community diabetes educator (CDE) staff the clinic. The dietitians offer nutritional counseling through a range of approaches, increasing patient choice.

Arne Sorenson is one of the two dietitians in the diabetes clinic. Based on his assessment of a patient's interest and ability levels, he incorporates additional educational materials to the commonly used (predating the 2005 revision) U.S. Department of Agriculture (USDA) food pyramid such as descriptive information on the carbohydrate content of foods and information on serving sizes.

Offering an alternative, dietician and diabetes educator Kibbe Conti uses a nutrition model that is currently catching the interest of tribes across the country. Based on her work with American Indian patients in South Dakota, Colorado, and California, Conti chooses a more culturally embedded nutrition model.

Initially, Conti worked with tribes and tribal members to develop a Four Winds Nutrition Model relevant to Plains Indians. That work, which we discuss in detail in the following section, has more recently formed the basis for a series of nutrition models reflecting the context, culture, and history of other tribal groups including a California Foodway model for Californian tribes and a model adapted for the Mandan, Hidatsa, and Arikara Nation.

Developing a Plains Indian Food Model

Seeking a more culturally relevant and effective nutritional model, Conti met with Lakota elders and a diabetic tribal member to discuss the possibility of developing a Plains Indian food model. Working together, the group created a food model linking healthy diets of early Plains Indians with currently available, and healthy, food choices.

They developed the Four Winds Nutrition Model, based on the medicine wheel, a Plains Indian symbol of healing, wisdom, and direction that her patients are familiar with, to help patients identify food groups, make healthier choices, and plan healthy meals. "The medicine wheel represents balance and is used by all Northern Plains tribes," Conti said. "Balance is recognized by the Lakota as an integral part of being human and requires care for physical, mental, and spiritual health."

This approach resulted in a model that Conti believes more accurately reflects Lakota and other Plains Indians' historic food choices. "For instance, their diet was not as grain-based as Northern Europeans may have been," Conti said. A quickly noticeable difference between the USDA's food pyramid and the Four Winds Nutrition Model is the removal of the dairy group as a distinct group because dairy was not historically in the Plains Indians' diet. The model does include dairy products throughout the quadrants. For instance, milk is included in the west quadrant as an unsweetened drink, and cheese is in the north quadrant as a good source of protein.

The Four Winds Nutrition Model

The quadrants of the medicine wheel, traditionally used by Plains Indians to represent the seasons, directions, and ages of life, are matched with four food categories: unsweetened beverages, good protein sources, fruits and vegetables, and starches (Exhibit 12.1).

Exhibit 12.1. Two Versions of the Four Winds Nutrition Model.

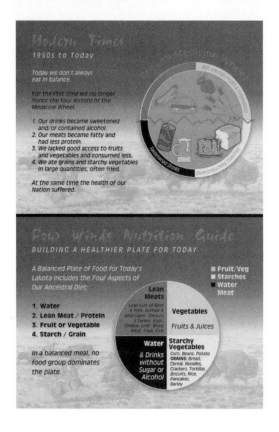

No category is meant to dominate another, resulting in a greater emphasis on protein and a lesser emphasis on carbohydrates than other nutrition guidelines often suggest.

The model tells the story of the diet transition of the Plains Indians from prereservation time to the present day in four parts. Each part, or version, of the narrative is centered on a modified medicine wheel. Across time, the food categories depicted by the wheel remain the same, but the foods themselves change throughout the sequence. The model confronts assumptions about what traditional foods and food preparation methods were. For instance, Conti explains that deep frying was not a traditional food preparation method and suggests healthy cooking options.

The first version of the wheel sets the stage for the narrative, placing the food groups into four quadrants of the medicine wheel. The second version teaches about the transition from a hunter-gather diet to a commodity food-based diet that developed when Plains Indians moved onto reservations. The third version shows unhealthy food and drink currently consumed on the reservation. The fourth, and final, version provides examples of how to choose healthy foods. The wheel is specific in naming food items that are available in the community.

Conti has recently adapted the Four Winds Wheel to a California Foodway model for Californian tribes and a model for the Mandan, Hidatsa, and Arikara Nation. Exhibit 12.2 depicts the four traditional food sources: cultivated foods, gathered foods, superior quality meats, and nourishing drink. Exhibit 12.3 depicts the events leading to the major shift away from traditional food sources caused by the construction of the Garrison Dam on the Missouri River. In the center is an image of tribal chairman George Gillette weeping at the signing of congressional legislation approving the dam's construction, which led to the eviction of native residents and the loss of approximately 150,000 acres of tribal homelands.

The model can be used in individual or group settings. At the end of each session, patients are given practice sheets with a four-quadrant medicine wheel to use in planning their own healthy breakfasts, lunches, and dinners. In her sessions, Conti has the patients plan several weeks of meals to ensure they are able to do so out of class.

"The desire is to challenge the participants," says Conti. She encourages them to think about identifying a food group when eating out: "Buffets are very popular in the area. They will be asked, 'If you're at a buffet what are you going to put on your plate?' Starch, for example, should only take up one-third of the plate, because West/unsweetened drink doesn't actually go on the plate."

Exhibit 12.2. Four Winds Nutrition Model Adapted for the Mandan, Hidatsa, and Arikara Nation: Traditional Food Sources.

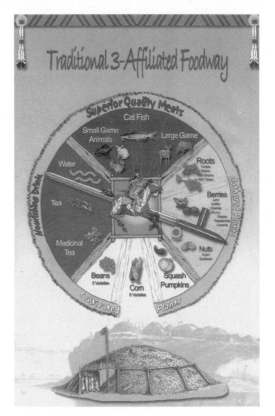

Applying the Nutrition Model

Maria Ramos, the diabetes program coordinator, hired Conti in 2002 to use the medicine wheel nutrition model in the diabetes clinic. Ramos tries to provide patients with a variety of nutrition models, one of which is the medicine wheel. "There are some ways that she may present [the Four Winds Nutrition Model] that might not be exactly what the American Dietetics Association says, but they're so similar that it allows people to change their eating habits by following this. If their blood sugars come down to normal, that's all we want," Ramos said.

Exhibit 12.3. Four Winds Nutrition Model Adapted for the Mandan, Hidatsa, and Arikara Nation: Loss of Tribal Homelands.

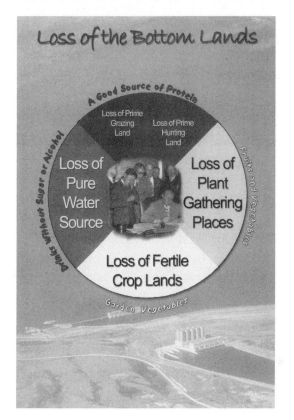

Ramos believes that the model presents a positive learning choice for her patients:

> I tell all my patients the same thing. I think they need to talk to her [Conti], they need to talk to our registered dietitian, and they also need to talk to our CDE. She [Conti] teaches the circle, he [Sorenson] teaches eat less food, eat less fat, eat less sugar, and our CDE teaches carb counting. So there are three different ways to look at nutrition from three different people. Everybody should

be able to look at them all, and all of them can be integrated because they all do the same thing. If people are
more comfortable with her approach, that's fine. If people are more comfortable with the "eat less food, eat less
fat," fine. If people want to sit down and start counting
carbs, that's fine too. We give them an option.

The Four Winds Nutrition Model is preferred by some of the
clinic's patients because it resonates with their lifestyles. "We have
some older Native Americans who do still eat some of the wild
game and stuff, so they like that part of the discussion. It's real simple for them to learn that way versus the carb counting versus calo-
rie counting and all the others. It's a more simple way of doing
approximately the same thing. But it's a little easier to understand,"
Ramos said. Alternatively, Native American youth can resist
attempts that place strong emphasis on historically traditional ways
of life. Thus, providing a balance of approaches reflecting the spectrum of individual patients' worldview is a more culturally responsive approach.

One of the reasons the model works is that it captures the interest of patients by resonating with their cultural contexts. The Four
Winds Nutrition Model is "not the usual sit down and say, okay, let's
talk about food," Ramos explained. "You can only eat this much,
this much, this much. She [Conti] doesn't start like that. She talks
about their history as a Native American and about how in the old
days we didn't have this and we didn't have that and about how
much healthier we were. That takes their interest, and everybody
knows that's how it was with our ancestors until all the Big Macs
came around and all that other stuff. Plus we had to work for our
living, physically work. Nobody just sat around and watched TV or
sat at a computer all day. People had their jobs; we were a roaming
nation. So everybody was always busy, and that's how she starts it,
and that catches people's interest."

Because of the cultural differences among Native American tribes across the United States, the model is meant for use with modification throughout the United States. Hugh Baker has led the Mandan, Hidatsa, and Arikara Nation in developing a tribe-specific food model based on a Mandan earth lodge: "I think we ought to be very specific and actually develop our own food model. Here you would first start with the tribal council and get them to adopt and approve the model and distribute it and work with the communities and get them to own some of it. You need to do that before you look for approval. We need to get support of the communities." In 2005 the USDA (2005b) began promoting an adjusted food pyramid that is less one-size-fits all as well.

Listening to the Community

Sometimes what seems like the best of ideas can have the worst outcomes. At other times, what some predict to fail creates a positive impact. Most important, efforts at prevention and care should be documented for their outcomes (see Chapter 13 on program evaluation). The challenge for program designers remains how to ensure effectiveness before program implementation and evaluating outcomes.

Charlene Johnson is the Crow Diabetes Project nutritionist in Crow Agency, Montana. She has tried a variety of healthy nutrition–promoting programs in her community. Some are more effective than others. For two years, she directed a health promotion and diabetes prevention program for community youth. During the first year, students were challenged to raise money for a walking path and obstacle course (the money raised was matched by the school district). The students organized a walk and earned well above their goal and decided to name the obstacle course after a Crow legend.

"They consulted a Crow elder on historic individuals who represented good physical ability," Johnson recounts. "He suggested a man by the name of Bear Coming Down Stream, who was a scout for a chief. Bear Coming Down Stream ran from Montana to Thermopolis, Wyoming [approximately 75 miles], and back within 24 hours to scout the enemy." After the course was built, it was named after Bear Coming Down Stream in a blessing ceremony.

The second year, Johnson had the students run a similar fundraiser, and they were even more successful. This money was used to put on a play based on the Crow legend. "The tribe's cultural coordinator wrote the play, which was performed by fifth graders. The play emphasized the physical prowess of Bear Coming Down Stream and talked about the diet of the Crow during his time," says Johnson.

During the play, a handout on physical activity, nutrition, and diabetes was distributed, and Crow women taught the students how to make dried meat. The program was well received in the community. It encouraged audience participation, made diabetes prevention learning fun and familiar, and promoted positive role models from within the community and the tribe's heritage.

Johnson shared with us the experience she gained during another community project in the Crow Agency that did not experience the same success. After hearing comments from patients that they would eat more vegetables if they had more money, knew how to grow vegetables, or had a rototiller for gardening, Johnson decided to promote gardening. She quickly received a small grant to teach gardening skills and provide rototilling, seeds, and starter plants to the community.

In a lesson we focus on in Chapter 13 on program evaluation, a carefully preconceived approach to program design and evaluation would have included a more thorough effort at understanding a community's views before embarking on a program. However, in this case, focus groups with community members were conducted only after the grant was received. This is far from unusual; many grants are awarded on what later turns out to be an incomplete understanding of the problem. In those instances, learning can still occur and future practices can be modified as appropriate, but efficiency is sacrificed.

In this case, the somewhat late-gathered focus group data made it clear that the gardening project was not entirely appropriate for the community. Those who were opposed to the project said that the Crow were historically hunter-gathers, not horticulturalists. Those individuals, based on their cultural history, see a negative association between gardening and the United States government's forcing the Crow to move onto reservations.

"Although they may have once gardened with the Mandan [another tribe], most gardening is associated with early reservation history," Johnson explained. "Settlers and the U.S. Army tried to get control of the Crow by encouraging them to grow crops." Those who opposed the gardening project cited that negative history or simply did not think it would fit their lives.

An unfortunate fit between a project as planned and the community it was hoped to work for does not necessarily mean there can be no positive impacts. Because the grant was already in hand, the diabetes project forged ahead with the gardening project but placed special emphasis on seeking to make the program attractive and feasible to community members. Their qualitative research made it clear that for the gardening project to be successful, it would require more than simply building a garden and providing the necessary tools and supplies.

To improve the original project design and transform the notion of gardening into one more acceptable to more community members, a tribal elder blessed each step of the project, from groundbreaking to setup of the greenhouse. In addition, the project incorporated plant choices that attempted to mirror traditional foods. They planted berries (a gatherer food) and sweetgrass (used in Crow ceremonies). The project also included classes on how to prepare the food being grown in the garden and hoped to entice community members by educating them on the benefits of the garden. However, the effort was not as well received as hoped.

Wrapping Up

Language is clearly not the sum total of culture, but at times the two are inseparable. Just as we strongly advocate that efforts at communication be crafted at the appropriate level of linguistic difficulty, they must also be crafted with the appropriate cultural characteristics in mind.

There is a richness and diversity in the approaches to the content and design of health interventions within Native American communities in the United States that this brief case study does not completely capture. As demonstrated in this case study, success is as likely to occur as a result of that bounty of approaches as it is from the specific culturally appropriate methods used to create that bounty. The diversity of approaches should reflect the rich variety in individuals, tribes, and communities.

However, just as is the case with linguistic skills, culture comes in a variety of shapes and sizes. While a one-size-fits all approach may be attractive to those who see an opportunity to lower costs, greater savings will ultimately emerge from designing programs that work. Culture, and by extension cultural literacy as a component of health literacy, is clearly part of a successful equation to improve health care, promote healthy decisions, and prevent unhealthy behaviors.

Common sense alone tells us that efforts grounded in the appropriate cultural context inherently have a better chance of success. Reducing cultural barriers makes it easier for individuals to receive, process, and understand information. Put simply, less cultural and linguistic translation is required. As we asserted at the outset of this case study, culture can be roughly thought of as an operating guide to common sense. The culture of medicine and health care should adopt a commonsense approach and consistently include culture as a component in the design of health care, health promotion, and health communication efforts.

Exercises

1. As a class, identify different cultural groups living within your community. Then review the list and determine what the distinctions among groups are based on; for example, race, history, ethnicity, or religion. Then develop a definition of culture based on that analysis. When defining *culture*, does one's own culture enter into the process? How? Does one culture become an unspoken norm, while others are distinguished from it?

2. Find health issues with prevalence, morbidity, or mortality rates that vary by cultural groups. Is there anything about culture that seems to make individuals more or less susceptible to the health problem? How would you address that?

3. Discuss the difference between biological and cultural determinants of disease. Do they often work in isolation? In tandem?

4. How would you design a research program to identify what cultural beliefs or practices influence decision making about healthy behaviors and health care? What cautions would you have to take?

13

Program Evaluation

World Education's Breast and Cervical Cancer Project

In homes, in hospitals and clinics, in schools and churches, and in community centers across the United States, people are teaching people to read, to write, and to work with numbers. In some cases, they are teaching about health and health care and trying to improve health literacy—one person, one class, one patient, and one day at a time. This work goes on far from the headlines and from made-for-TV dramas, often without notice or reward by the very systems and society they support. These are the people and places on the front lines of progress.

How do we know whether these efforts succeed or fail? How can we make less effective efforts better? How do we learn from the programs that work? The answers can be found through effective program evaluation, which is often unwelcome news to program managers and accountants, who see only an extra cost in an era of ever-tightening budgets.

This case study addresses two fundamental questions facing health literacy practitioners on a daily basis. First, how can we determine which efforts fail, which succeed, and how that happened? Second, and of equal if not greater importance, how can we

---

This chapter was prepared with the assistance of Sabrina Kurtz-Rossi, Sally Waldron, and Judy Titzel of World Education.

design better programs to improve health literacy? As an example, we draw on World Education's Health Education and Adult Literacy: Breast and Cervical Cancer Project (HEAL:BCC) funded by the Centers for Disease Control and Prevention (Exhibit 13.1).

Adult Basic Education and Health Literacy

In a too often underrewarded and underrecognized effort, thousands of adult basic education (ABE) and English for speakers of other languages (ESOL) programs throughout the United States address the educational needs of millions of adults with low functional literacy. The adults who enroll in ABE or ESOL classes, an estimated 4 million during 2001, are also those most often at greater health risk, including those with low income, or low educational attainment, or perhaps immigrants with limited English language skills.

Personal and group characteristics such as race, ethnicity, culture, and socioeconomic status greatly influence access to health infor-

Exhibit 13.1. Logo for the HEAL:BCC Project.

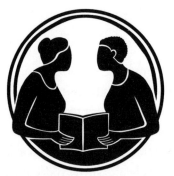

Health Education and Adult Literacy
HEAL: Breast & Cervical Cancer

A project of World Education in cooperation with the Centers for Disease Control and Prevention

---

Why Evaluate?

Evaluation seeks to produce evidence that can be used to make something better. Among the many things that do not define evidence are these (Perkins, Simnett & Wright, 1999):

- Saying, "I've done this for 25 years, and I know!"

- A set of morals

- Casual conversations

- Anecdotal information

- A brainstorming session

- Continuing the status quo

- Arguments in defense of past actions

- An opinion or value

- Something only Ph.D.s can gather

- A new idea that seems good

---

mation, understanding and use of that information, and health outcomes. While identifying and addressing each of these contributing characteristics is a daunting task for the health care system, ABE and ESOL classes are well suited to address and assess learners' individual needs. Literacy programs are an important environment in which to introduce and develop health literacy skills by infusing health into the literacy curriculum, effectively tailoring information to the students' health literacy abilities and real life needs.

The purpose of adult education is to equip learners with the knowledge and skills they need to access information, take independent action, and continue to learn throughout their lives

(Hohn, 1997). Adult literacy education focuses on enabling learners to become active participants in meeting their life needs. This aim is best achieved by broadening the focus from individual learners' skills to approaches connecting literacy to the social, historical, political, cultural, and personal situations where people use their skills (Fingeret, 1990, 1992).

Especially from the perspective put forth in this book—that health literacy is a rich resource that enables individuals to productively apply information to address new health issues that emerge—efforts to improve health literacy are clearly a good fit with the mission of ABE and ESOL education. In the adult literacy system, there is a growing awareness of the connections between low literacy and poor health and the need to work collaboratively with health care professionals. The same is true in reverse.

Working together, the health and adult literacy systems can begin to address the depth and scope of interconnected issues that affect individual and community health. A central challenge is how to document programs that work, improve efforts that are less successful, and share best practices with others.

Targeting Breast and Cervical Cancer

Fundamentally, this case demonstrates the potential of introducing health and health literacy into ABE and ESOL programs. However, we explicitly draw on the experience of the HEAL:BCC program to highlight the critical importance of program evaluations.

The HEAL:BCC Project, which began in 1998, was built on three years of formative evaluation conducted by Rima Rudd of the Harvard School of Public Health and earlier World Education projects. A goal was to better meet the needs of ABE teachers and their students. Rudd designed the initial curriculum framework and approach. Cathy Coyne of the West Virginia University School of Medicine designed the evaluation to look at the impact of introducing breast and cervical cancer health content in ABE and ESOL classes. Coyne feels that "evaluation is an essential component of the program development process. Without adequately evaluating a new program before it is disseminated for use in the community, a program may be implemented with tremendous effort on the part of teachers and learners without having the intended results."

Program evaluation is an activity that comes in many shapes and sizes. An ideal evaluation design produces reliable, valid, and useful results and is affordable. When well designed and performed, evaluation can positively influence a program's formative design, implementation, outcomes, and sustainability.

Specific issues we address in this case study are:

- The functions, goals, means, and limitations of program evaluation

- The choice between qualitative and quantitative approaches

- The importance and role of applying theory to program design and evaluation

- The impact of a well-planned and well-evaluated health literacy component in an ABE and ESOL program

- The challenge of measuring health literacy

The HEAL:BCC development, pilot activities, full-scale implementation, and evaluation was a systematic and thorough effort to study and collect both qualitative and quantitative outcome data to evaluate the effectiveness of introducing specific health content into ABE classes in the United States. The project promoted the diffusion of information about breast and cervical cancer early detection and screening through ABE and ESOL classes. The program was designed to meet the health information and skills development needs of adults with limited health literacy. A primary goal was to increase screening and early detection for breast and cervical cancer among low-income and minority women with less than a high school education.

Beginning in the 1990s, lessons learned from World Education's programs with women in Nepal and India that integrated health and family planning information with basic literacy skill development were applied to developing World Education's U.S. literacy programs.

In 1992, World Education's Massachusetts Cancer Education and Literacy Initiative (ELI) was funded by the U.S. National Cancer Institute to develop resources for low-literacy adults on breast and cervical cancer. ELI used a participatory approach to curriculum development so that students, ABE and ESOL teachers, a literacy curriculum specialist, and health professionals worked together to identify and address critical issues related to cancer education and early detection and to build strategies for overcoming barriers.

A core product of ELI, *The Breast and Cervical Cancer Sourcebook*, was subsequently field-tested by teachers throughout New England as a component of World Education's Health Education and Adult Literacy (HEAL) Project in 1994. HEAL promoted use of the *Sourcebook* across New England and included a teacher training program that helped teachers examine their fears about addressing cancer, prepared them to bring a variety of innovative health lessons into their classrooms, and supported teachers and students designing learning materials together.

HEAL curriculum presented a common challenge to teachers, summed up by Pat Connors: "I signed on to be one of the New England field test teachers for HEAL, and I was nearly paralyzed with fear when I initially started. I had no idea of how to present explicit information about breast and cervical cancer. HEAL was asking me to explore my fears and take an important step forward in my teaching." We have found this to be a common concern in the adult literacy world: practitioners who feel unprepared to tackle health or environmental issues as part of their content.

A major product of HEAL was the *Breast and Cervical Cancer Resource Kit*, which was designed to help teachers introduce breast and cervical cancer information into literacy classes by providing articles, books, posters, videos, and a wide array of other tools and curriculum templates. The kit, reviewed by health and literacy experts and piloted by more than 200 teachers in 16 states, increased teachers' cancer-related knowledge and skills while simultaneously providing materials that both teachers and students could use in the classroom.

HEAL:BCC development, pilot activities, full-scale implementation, and evaluation took place within adult learning centers, a preestablished network accessed and generally trusted by the students, who were often minority, low-income, and low-literacy women. Components of the HEAL:BCC model include a center-wide orientation; training for teachers who will implement the curriculum; an adult learning center resource box of materials; the HEAL:BCC Curriculum (Exhibit 13.2); student materials including the HEAL:BCC *Word List* and *Passport to Health* (Exhibit 13.3); technical assistance and support; linkages with local breast and cervical cancer screening providers; and a final project event. HEAL:BCC focuses on the forms of cancer that have extremely high rates of mortality among the target population.

In the earlier ELI and HEAL programs, agreements to use the materials were made with individual teachers, whereas in the HEAL:BCC program, agreements were made with centers. The result was that more than one teacher would be teaching the curriculum so that individual teachers would be less likely to work in isolation. In addition, the HEAL:BCC effort explicitly included linking adult education centers with sources of health information and health care in their own community.

"If you bring health topics up in the classroom, especially ones that encourage screening and early detection, you have to offer a place were learners can go for health services," said Sabrina Kurtz-Rossi, HEAL:BCC director. "While establishing a connection

Exhibit 13.2. HEAL:BCC Curriculum.

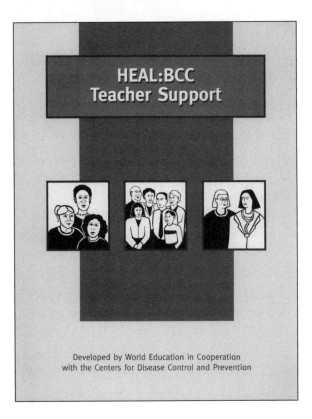

between a local adult learning center and clinic or hospital can sometimes be challenging, it is critical to the success of the program."

The HEAL:BCC project took place in early 2001, in partnership between World Education and 17 adult learning centers in five states. In Florida, all the centers were located in Hillsborough County. In Virginia, centers were located in four counties across the state. In New York, all participating centers were located in Manhattan. In the combined Rhode Island and Massachusetts site, three centers were located in Providence, Rhode Island, and one in southeastern Massachusetts.

Exhibit 13.3. HEAL:BCC *Word List* and *Passport to Health*.

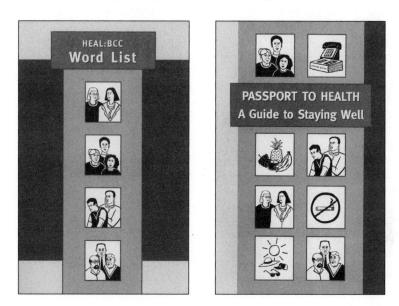

What Is Evaluation?

According to the American Evaluation Association (http://www. eval.org), the many and diverse approaches to evaluation share the common ground of aspiring "to construct and provide the best possible information that might bear on the value of whatever is being evaluated" (American Evaluation Association, 1994). Having a subject to evaluate, however, is only a first step in the process. A next step involves deciding what exactly is to be evaluated about the subject. Leading evaluation methodologist Michael Q. Patton identifies a number of potential foci for evaluation: implementation, outcomes, process, program comparisons, development over time, individual outcomes, logic models and theories of action, prevention, and evaluability (Patton, 2003).

Evaluation can:

- Justify the program to funders and management

- Provide evidence of success

- Document a need for additional resources

- Indicate areas requiring program modification and improvement

- Increase organizational understanding of individual programs

- Encourage cooperative ventures with other organizations

- Facilitate the sharing of best practices

At the most fundamental level, programs and projects tend to have formative stages, where the program is being developed; implementation stages, where the program is beginning; process stages, when the program is ongoing; and outcome stages, what the program makes change. Each of these stages can be a focus of evaluation. Focusing on different stages produces different information and meets different needs.

Outline of an Evaluation Process

1. Define program goals.

2. Define setting and intended audiences.

3. Construct a theoretical framework.

4. Develop indicators.

5. Select methodologies and the research design.

6. Collect data (for example, baseline, progress, and outcomes).

7. Interpret data.

8. Prepare the evaluation report.

9. Disseminate the evaluation report.

The focus of an evaluation, from implementation to outcomes, should reflect the goals of the effort being evaluated and the desired uses and impacts of the evaluation. For example, if a program's ultimate goal is to increase knowledge, an evaluation that focuses on measuring health status or implementation will have less relevance than an evaluation that focuses on what knowledge was acquired. Similarly, if a program wants to learn how it differed from other efforts in order to make future adjustments, an evaluation that looked only at outcomes would have less to offer than one that focused on formative, implementation, and process stages.

HEAL:BCC Implementation and Evaluation

In addition to formative and outcome evaluation, the HEAL:BCC program included a process evaluation component. "Throughout the HEAL:BCC project, feedback from teachers and learners played an important role in the development of the materials and model," Kurtz-Rossi said. For example, a valuable lesson was learned during the early piloting of the curriculum: "Students told us that they wanted to see phonetic spellings in the Word List. Adopting that early suggestion from students greatly improved the Word List and made it one of the most popular final products of the program."

The HEAL:BCC evaluation documented significant changes in areas of knowledge gain among students as well as behavior change: the number of women who reported having a Pap test and the frequency that students suggested screenings to sisters, friends, classmates, and coworkers. One student reported, "It's a good program. I didn't know a lot of things, and I found [out] about them. Now I'm just telling whoever I know."

How did all this successful teaching, learning, and healthy behavior change come about for the students, the teachers and centers, and health literacy researchers and practitioners? Certainly the years of development by World Education and its partners deserve

much of the credit. That history informed the application of communication and education theories within the realities of ABE and
ESOL classrooms to create a successful program design and evaluation framework.

Mission Statements and Theory

Theory is a guide for a researcher's reasoning about how to evaluate a program's claims and goals. The task of choosing a theoretical
framework and accompanying methodology for program design and
evaluation requires a clear and shared understanding of the program's goals that should be in the mission statement. Often, however, a program's mission statement is a collection of abstract terms
that lends little to evaluation efforts or, in fact, the program's day-
to-day operations. In those cases, a set of goals must be developed
that reflects exactly what a program hopes to accomplish. That must
occur before a successful evaluation can begin.

If the expertise, or agreement, does not exist within the program
to perform the tasks of identifying appropriate goals and selecting
theories on which to base evaluation, outside consultants or assistance should be sought. The expense of appropriate evaluation is
well justified by the benefits to the program since a primary goal of
evaluation should be the production of knowledge usable to improve performance. In addition, governments increasingly require
evaluations of publicly funded projects, as exemplified by the Government Performance Results Act in the United States and the
Research Assessment Exercise in the United Kingdom, and there
are established corporate governance and evaluation codes in the
private sector as well.

Initially the HEAL:BCC program relied on the theory of diffusion of innovations to provide structure for program development,
implementation, and evaluation. But through experience and insights gained during the early phases of the program, it became apparent that the diffusion theory did not account for all the factors
affecting the program's success and failure. As a result, HEAL:BCC

employed an ecological model with the diffusion of innovations theory to build a theoretical framework that better matched its experiences in adult education.

The final choices of theoretical frameworks reflect the three main goals of the program: to (1) increase breast and cervical cancer screening and early detection, (2) encourage "healthful action" related to breast and cervical cancer, and (3) promote healthful action within the community through improvements in the lay referral system.

For the first, and perhaps the most straightforward, goal, the diffusion of innovations takes the lead. The theory predicts that attributes of each person, such as attitudes and beliefs, are related to the uptake of a new practice or idea and that change agents can facilitate the diffusion of this new practice or idea throughout the community. The evaluation measured knowledge and attitudes about breast and cervical cancer screening and early detection among adult learners before and after the program and whether learners shared what they had learned with others in their community. The evaluation also included a measure of the number of female learners who obtained a Pap test, mammogram, or clinical breast exam before and after the HEAL:BCC curriculum was introduced. If the program resulted in the predicted impacts, individuals who experienced positive changes in knowledge and attitudes toward breast and cervical cancer screening would also be more likely to have undergone or plan to undergo screening, which is exactly what happened.

An ecological theory of health and health behavior change predicts that if the environment was supportive of learning and behavior change, then that change would be more likely to be adopted. Focusing on the ecological model, the evaluation included measures of activity in support of the HEAL:BCC curriculum within the environment of the adult learning centers that participated in the program. Specific indicators included factors such as the number of bulletin boards in the center displaying information about breast and cervical cancer and the number and frequency of center-wide activities related to the curriculum.

Employing both theories as guides corresponds with the belief that the overall environment in learning centers does impact the success of efforts but also that individual champions of an idea and the characteristics of individual teachers and learners clearly matter as well. As a result, the evaluation was able to explicitly incorporate baseline, process, and outcome measures for impacts and attributes in individuals as well as in the overall environment of the learning center.

For practitioners and educators involved in their own program and evaluations, the lesson is not to use the same theories that HEAL:BCC selected but to employ appropriate theories as a framework for designing and evaluating programs. In other instances—given the wide variety of environments and specific goals possible (for example, to improve health status, improve knowledge, improve basic skills, or improve abilities to interact with the health care system)—other theories will prove more productive and appropriate.

Marrying Theory with Practice

A theoretical framework provides the scaffolding on which program strategies and evaluation indicators are built. The framework outlines the areas of action and evaluation, but there remains a choice of which individual indicators to select.

Evidence of the application of the diffusion model comes from Kurtz-Rossi, who said, "In Connecticut, Florida, Rhode Island, and Virginia HEAL:BCC students organized health fairs at their centers and invited their relatives and friends to attend. They took what they had learned in class and passed it on to others. We heard reports of non-HEAL:BCC students going for breast and cervical cancer screening, but a major challenge of the HEAL:BCC evaluation was capturing this broader impact."

Given the inherent difficulty of measuring a multidomain construct such as health literacy and the current lack of an ideal measure,

Measuring Health Literacy:
An Effort in Development

There are two popular measures used by researchers and practitioners to measure health literacy: the Rapid Estimate of Adult Literacy in Medicine (REALM) and the Test of Functional Health Literacy in Adults (TOFHLA). This is an area where more development is needed as, at best, the current measures address only some aspects of the functional domain of health literacy and fall far short of providing evaluators with a complete assessment of an individual's true health literacy.

The REALM consists of 66 health- or medical-related words arranged in progressive difficulty and can generally be completed in two minutes. It does not address numeracy skills or any of the more complex concepts contained within many health literacy definitions, including the one put forth in this book.

The TOFHLA is available in English and Spanish, large print, and a shortened version (S-TOFHLA). According to the developers, "The S-TOFHLA appears to have good reliability (internal consistency) and is a valid measure of patients' ability to read the materials they are likely to encounter in the health care setting (i.e. health literacy)" (Baker, Williams, Parker, Gazmararian, & Nurss, 1999, p. 38).

While perhaps the best measures currently available, the REALM and TOFHLAs nevertheless do not address the multiple domains of health literacy explicated in this book. In a recent review of the field, Rogers, Ratzan, and Payne (2001) concluded that "the ideal measure of health literacy would be short and quick, include both numeracy as well as reading ability, and also deal with the ability to think critically about the medical/health system. Furthermore, an ideal measure would not be offensive or embarrassing to patients. Our review of literature did not disclose a health literacy measure that met all of these criteria, so further effort is needed to develop improved measures" (p. 2184).

HEAL:BCC evaluators instead focused on what they felt were the most predictive aspects of health literacy in relation to the behavior changes the program was trying to effect. In the end, the evaluation measured change in knowledge among adult learners about key facts and vocabulary related to breast and cervical cancer prevention and early screening as a surrogate for a more complete measure of health literacy.

All of these indicators, and many more we have not delineated in this case study, were assessed within the classrooms and adult education centers both before and after the curriculum was used. In addition, some indicators were measured during the progress of using the curriculum in the classrooms. These issues lead us to the next important topic of this case study, the design of an evaluation.

Choosing an Evaluation Design

Deciding how to design an evaluation is performed in parallel with the choice of individual indicators and the theoretical framework. Those choices are not independent: each choice of design, theory, and indicators mutually influences the others. In medical research, in particular with the growing emphasis on evidence-based medicine, the gold standard for evidence is the systematic review of randomized control trials. Observational studies are usually deemed to be lesser sources of evidence, although research has demonstrated that observational studies "do not systematically overestimate the magnitude of the effects of treatment as compared with those in randomized, controlled trials on the same topic" (Concato, Shah, & Horwitz, 2000, p. 1887).

For most health literacy, health promotion, and health education programs, an experimental design such as the randomized control trial is impractical, ineffective, or beset with ethical problems (Webb, 1999). A randomized control trial, in the most basic form, consists of at least two randomly selected groups, one of which receives the intervention and one of which does not in a setting designed to prevent, or limit, any outside influences on the hypoth-

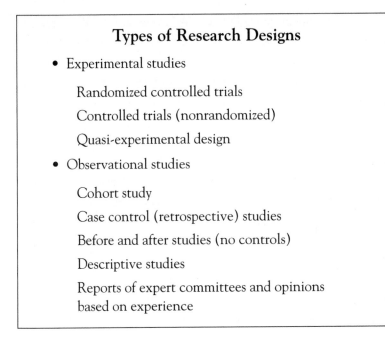

Types of Research Designs

- Experimental studies

  Randomized controlled trials

  Controlled trials (nonrandomized)

  Quasi-experimental design

- Observational studies

  Cohort study

  Case control (retrospective) studies

  Before and after studies (no controls)

  Descriptive studies

  Reports of expert committees and opinions
  based on experience

esized effect. This design presents the following problems (Perkins et al., 1999):

- It is impossible to ethically or practically separate individuals from their cultural contexts, and from each other, in such a way as to ensure that the intervention was the sole influence.

- A host of ethical problems emerge when considering denying individuals access to useful and relevant knowledge about their health.

- Random controlled trials are limited in their effectiveness to measure complex interventions such as those employed in making individual and social change.

- Random controlled trials focus on outcomes at the expense of gathering knowledge about process and implementation.

These difficulties can place evaluators in a bind between the gold standard of evidence within the biomedical community and the reality of program implementation and evaluation. As a result, it is increasingly common to encounter a quasi-experimental design in evaluation of social programs, and that is the choice the HEAL:BCC evaluators made.

A quasi-experimental research design is one that has some elements of the classic experimental design but may lack a pretest, or a control group, use more than two groups, or define groups based on locality rather than as individuals. In general, quasi-experimental designs surrender some of the rigid control of a classic experimental design but are often better suited to the realities of practice (Patton, 2003).

Most important, the research design that programs select should produce results that are the most relevant and useful. That may mean that a quasi-experimental design with quantitative research methods is used, or it may mean that the best choice is a descriptive study based on entirely qualitative research methods.

The HEAL:BCC choice of a quasi-experimental design was primarily dictated by the fact that the groups were not randomly selected or matched but were based on the locations of the participating adult education centers. Also, although the design did include a control group, many of the differences between the centers that offered the curriculum and the adult education center that did not offer the curriculum could not be controlled for by the research design. Those variables may well have impacted the outcomes of the study. That does imply that the HEAL:BCC evaluation was of less than optimal quality from a research purist's perspective, as the changes recorded in the pre- and postmeasures may not be entirely accounted for by the HEAL:BCC curriculum. Nonetheless, the strength of the quasi-experimental design in this case is that it allowed evaluators to maintain the highest control possible given the reality of the situation.

According to Coyne, the HEAL:BCC evaluator, "There are several limitations to the study of the HEAL:BCC project. A significant strength however, is that it was conducted in a real-life setting, that is, in existing adult learning center classrooms, and implemented by real teachers, not just staff hired by the project. Evaluation of the project within this type of setting increases the generalizability of the findings."

Choosing a Quantitative or Qualitative Approach

Quantitative research is used to gather information by asking a large number of people a set of identical questions. Results are generally expressed in numerical terms (for example, "35 percent are aware of X and 65 percent are not," or "socioeconomic status accounted for 28 percent of the variance of the outcome measure with a p value below .05") and rely on statistical methods to determine validity and reliability. If the respondents are a representative random sample, quantitative data can be used to draw conclusions about an intended audience as a whole. Quantitative research is useful for measuring the extent to which knowledge, attitude, or behavior is prevalent in an intended audience (Bryman, 1992; Ragin, 1994; Lofland & Lofland, 1995).

Qualitative research is used to gather reactions and impressions, usually by engaging the participants in discussion. Results are often not described numerically or used to make generalizations about the larger population. Research design methods such as gathering and comparing (triangulating) data from different sources are used to determine validity and reliability. Qualitative research is useful for understanding why people react the way they do and for understanding additional ideas, issues, concerns, and how they may be framing an issue. Qualitative data are not used to test hypotheses; rather, they are more often used as a first step in the research process geared toward constructing hypotheses that can then be tested by quantitative methodologies.

Some researchers value qualitative data and others quantitative data. We recommend selecting the approach that best promises to meet the needs of the assessment, the program, and, most important, the people the program was established to help.

The HEAL:BCC evaluation employed both quantitative and qualitative approaches. Quantitative methods were mainly employed in the pre- and posttests to evaluate the extent and nature of change in the students, teachers, and adult education centers. Qualitative methods were employed to focus on the process of implementation, make alterations and additions to the program as needed while in progress, and provide a broader context to the quantitative data.

A marriage of types of data can be most helpful if balanced appropriately. For example, Coyne was initially concerned that they were placing too much of a burden on teachers with demands for

---

Reliability and Validity

Reliability and validity are two basic properties of empirical measurements. *Reliability* refers to the likelihood that consistent results will be obtained if the measure, test, or experiment is repeated. *Validity* refers to the agreement between the indicator and the concept it is supposed to reflect.

For example, we can easily imagine a measure, or indicator, of health literacy that produces consistent results, which is to say it seems to be reliable. However, the measure may actually be measuring something other than health literacy, like just the ability to read or the amount of medically related scientific knowledge an individual possesses. That measure would be highly reliable but not high on validity (Carmines & Zeller, 1979).

feedback and quantitative information: "The challenge in this evaluation was to select methods that will not impose an excessive burden on the learners and teachers yet will provide the information needed to assess whether the program had its intended results."

During the process evaluation stage, which mainly relied on qualitative methods, they learned that the teachers were not put out by the information requests. All was not perfect, however, as the process feedback also informed HEAL:BCC program designers that the center-wide assessment tool needed to be made available in Spanish as well. As a result, the questions were translated. In essence, the qualitative results not only informed the evaluators but also helped refine the quantitative tools during the process of the evaluation itself.

Lessons Learned from the Evaluation

Valuable lessons were learned about incorporating specific health information into an ABE curriculum and documented by the evaluation of HEAL:BCC:

• Process evaluation and qualitative results show that teachers need institutional support to teach sensitive health topics in their classrooms. Materials and supports developed by the ELI and HEAL projects focused on teachers; HEAL:BCC was designed to engage entire programs and included center-wide orientation, teacher training, ongoing support, and connections to local breast and cervical cancer screening sites.

• Both the ELI and HEAL projects developed open-ended materials for teachers and adult learners to select from, adapt, and use. During the HEAL project, teachers reported that developing specific lesson plans on cancer education was challenging, even given substantial resource materials. As a result, the HEAL:BCC project developed a core curriculum that teachers could follow that integrated health content and literacy skills.

• During HEAL:BCC, teachers and students preferred a core curriculum that integrated health and literacy skills in no more than 15 or 16 lessons. A longer curriculum was less likely to be used in its entirety.

• Given institutional support and a curriculum and resources, teachers did not need intensive face-to-face support as they were implementing the HEAL:BCC curriculum. But process evaluation revealed that they did need background information, breast and cervical cancer contacts, and additional resources. As a result, a teacher support document was developed.

• Although the HEAL:BCC curriculum was originally designed for intermediate through advanced ABE and ESOL classes, center-wide evaluation found that ESOL classes at all levels wanted to participate in HEAL:BCC. Teachers needed to adjust the curriculum for students at different English-language proficiency levels and discuss cultural health issues, so instructional and cultural notes were added to the curriculum.

• Students wanted health resources that would help them educate others within their communities; therefore student resources such as the HEAL:BCC *Word List* and *Passport to Health* were developed.

• Self-administered quantitative and qualitative questionnaires can be used in the classroom, with the assistance of the teacher, to collect information about health knowledge gain. Teachers did not find it burdensome to administer pre- and postsurveys, although they recommended native-language surveys for non-English speakers and a translated word list for teachers to use when administering the English-language questionnaire.

Wrapping Up

This chapter, employing the HEAL:BCC program and evaluation as a core example, has highlighted several important lessons about program evaluation:

- Begin planning and conducting evaluation before the start of the program.

- Develop evaluation indicators that reflect the program's design and goals.

- Employ an appropriate theoretical framework to the design of evaluation. Match theory to practice.

- The goal of evaluation should be to produce useful and relevant information.

- Evaluation, when done correctly, is well worth additional program expense.

Exercises

1. After providing program materials of an example of an effort to improve health literacy, educate people about a health issue, or promote a healthy behavior, have students individually write down what they think the goals of the program are. Then discuss these points:

   Does everyone agree on the goals?

   What are the causes of any disagreements that emerge?

   What indicators or measures could you develop to see if the example met its goals?

   What theories do you think the program was informed by, if any?

   How would you go about designing an evaluation to see if the program met its goals?

2. You are brought in to evaluate a children's after-school weight-loss program attended by 60 children and run by a school-based nurse and health educator. The approach is to use a computer interactive program. The main goals of the

program are to help children feel supported by one another, learn principles of better eating habits, make healthier food choices during the school day, and bring information about good food choices home to their families. How would you go about designing this evaluation? What indicators are most important? Why?

14

Guidelines for Advancing Health Literacy

Advancing an individual's or a public's health literacy should be a central function of health promotions, education, and communication. In order for health promotions to get the job done, they have to be linguistically and culturally appropriate and have to build on the types and degree of literacy the consumer already has—fundamental, scientific, civic, and cultural—to develop the health literacy skills they need to take part in the discourse about health. The following guidelines are derived from the major points made in the previous chapters. They are the product of our own research and clinical experience as well as the research of others.

In the guidelines, we use the term *text* to refer to written, spoken, and visual texts. A text can be as short as a slogan or as long as a booklet or book, as compact as one graphic symbol or a full advertisement or poster, a spoken one-line direction or full-length radio announcement. In other words, a text is any print, spoken, visual, or auditory message that coheres and is meaningful.

When there are guidelines for a specific type of text, we indicate this. As with any other guidelines, there is no one right way to create health promotion and health education programs and messages that meet the needs of a particular target audience. Awareness of people's needs and literacy skills along with good common sense will take you a long way in applying health literacy principles to your communication. As an old medical school dictum says, when you hear the drumbeat of hooves, think horses, not zebras.

Guideline 1: General

All health promotions, whether an individual message or full campaign, should follow these general guidelines:

- Know your audience.

- Use initial and in-process field research methods to inform your approach.

- Collaborate with your target audiences to cooperatively write and create materials and messages.

- Field-test using a combination of observations, in-depth reader-listener response interviews, focus groups, and panels.

- Budget time, money, and personnel for the entire effort.

- Evaluate the impact of your communication campaign periodically.

Being clear about the main goals of a communication is vital. Too often the sender wants to include too many different messages in one communication. The resulting long, complicated communications are hard to read or listen to and harder to remember. Often, in order to keep the language simple, messages become disjointed, lack cohesion and logic, and are hard to read.

Use these questions to reflect on and determine the goals of your communication:

- Is it to inform or educate, or both?

- Is it to gather information through a survey or questionnaire?

- Is it intended to produce action or a change of behavior?

- Will it be used with mediation; that is, will someone assist the patient or public?

- What medium or technology will be used?

- What types of health literacy are required? What domain dominates the message?

- What health literacy skills will the message help develop?

- How culturally appropriate is this message?

- To whom is it tailored?

- What does it require the target audience to understand about science, health, civic, and cultural factors?

- Will this message be repeated and reinforced in any way?

- How will you know if the message is understood?

- How will you involve the audience early and often in the design of your messages or campaigns?

- Have you capitalize on spoken and written competencies?

- How will this advance a person's health literacy?

Know your audience. There is no one magic bullet that will tell you precisely what a person or public needs to know about health and how that information is best conveyed. There are health literacy assessment tools and health belief surveys, but as any experienced professional will agree, there is no substitute for listening and looking carefully at what people say and how they make meaning. The task of identifying the health literacy and health information and modality preferences of an audience will most often be limited by time, budget, and expertise.

The best way to understand the language and literacy needs of an audience is through a combination of quantitative and qualitative research. Qualitative research—observations, interviews, and group discussions (focus groups and panels)—is especially useful for exploration and discovery (Ragin, 1994; Lofland & Lofland, 1995). Potential beneficiaries of qualitative research are participants (not seen as "subjects"). They are intimately involved in creating and revising the research materials through their direct contact with the writer or message developer (McTaggart, 1997; Zarcadoolas et al., 2001). (See the Chapter 13 case study on evaluation.)

Quantitative methods can be effectively used to interact with large audiences, gain their perceptions and responses, and then translate the information gathered back into useful and relevant concepts (see discussion of field testing later in this chapter).

Use the appropriate research methods, discussed in Chapter 13, to ask the following sorts of questions about an audience's health literacy:

- What is their spoken language ability?

- What barriers do they face in reading this text?

- What is the level of vocabulary, sentence structure, and other important text elements in your message or communication?

- What assumptions does this message make, and does the consumer share enough knowledge to comprehend the most important parts of it?

- How relevant is the message?

- How trustworthy is the messenger?

- How culturally appropriate is the message?

Guideline 2: Vocabulary

Use clear and understandable vocabulary. Most people do not understand technical terms or jargon (see the examples in Exhibit 14.1). It is also important to define and clarify all new or difficult words within a text (see Exhibit 14.2).

Simplify vocabulary and define all complex words on the page. Do not rely on a glossary. It interrupts reading and comprehension, and many readers do not use it. Use one-word alternatives or simple phrases.

Exhibit 14.1. Example: Hard-to-Read Vocabulary and Easy-to-Read Vocabulary.

Hard to Read	Easy to Read
• Eligible	• Can join, can receive
• Respond	• Answer, send
• Receive	• Get
• Exempt	• You don't have
• Inhale	• Breathe in
• Inoculation	• Shot
• Evacuate	• Leave
• Potable	• Safe to drink

Exhibit 14.2. Example: Defining Words in the Text.

- This is an official notice. An official notice is a formal notice and it means you must answer this letter by _____ (date). [The second sentence defines the term "notice" in the first sentence.]

- We did not approve your application for TANF cash assistance because you did not provide (did not give) us the information we asked for. [The synonym is in parentheses.]

- City officials will go on radio to tell you if you have to evacuate (leave) your homes. [The difficult word is defined in parentheses on first use and then can be used throughout the rest of the text as the primary word.]

Avoid legal terminology unfamiliar to your audience—for example:

> *Instead of*: "I declare that I have read and understand the application."
>
> *Try*: "If I sign my name below, this means that I read and I understand this application."

If you must use technical words (for instance, if you will be talking about a certain topic repeatedly and over time with consumers), normalize (make familiar) and teach these words or terms (Exhibit 14.3).

Make the "skip-and-guess strategy" easier for readers or listeners:

> Example: Today the doctor gave you a medication. You must take the pill the doctor gave you twice a day.

Exhibit 14.3. Example: Normalizing.

Instead of	*Try*
"Utility disruption": Although infrequent, utility service disruptions—power outages, water or gas supply emergencies, and telephone service interruptions—are not unprecedented. [New York City Office of Emergency Management, n.d., para. 1].	"The power goes out": During a storm you can have disruptions in your utilities—no power, or problems with water, gas, and telephone. If you have a problem with your utilities . . .
"I declare under penalty of perjury that the answers I have given . . ."	"I know that if I do not tell the truth on this application I am breaking the law."

Source: For the utility disruption example: New York City Office of Emergency Management (n.d., para. 1).

Even if the reader does not understand the word *medication*, reading the second sentence will help the reader make a good guess that "medication" refers to a pill.

Guideline 3: Sentences

Sentence length and sentence complexity are key factors in how understandable information is. They both affect readability, but they are not the only important factors:

- Long sentences should be simple sentences that use simple conjunctions: *and, but, or.* In the example in Exhibit 14.4, the revised sentence is very long but not complex. It is a series of simple sentences conjoined, that is, joined by *and, or,* and *but.*
- Write sentences in which the main noun and verb are not far away from each other (that is, not interrupted by phrases and clauses).
- When you use relative clauses, make sure the referent is clear. Avoid relative clauses that seriously interrupt a simple (noun + verb + modifier) sentence.
- Unpack complex sentences. Divide them into simpler sentences, but make and preserve cohesive ties (Exhibit 14.5).

Exhibit 14.4. Example: Revising Groups of Sentences.

Hard to Read	*Easy to Read*
Going to the emergency room is a covered expense if you are experiencing conditions that are so serious that any reasonable person could assume that these conditions are life threatening. Acceptable conditions include: trouble breathing, heavy bleeding, or chest pain.	When should you go to the emergency room? You should go to the emergency room if you are bleeding heavily, or if you are having trouble breathing, or if there is a danger that you could die.

Exhibit 14.5. Example: Complex Versus Simple Sentences.

Complex Sentences That Are Hard to Read	*Simpler Sentences That Are Easier to Read*
Getting prenatal care as soon as you think you are pregnant and going to your health care provider for prenatal care throughout your pregnancy are the best things you can do to have a healthy baby.	The two most important things you can do to have a healthy baby: (1) Go see your doctor/nurse as soon as you think you are pregnant. (2) Visit your doctor/nurse all through your pregnancy.

Exhibit 14.6. Example: Varying Sentence Length and Complexity.

Use a complex sentence only when there are simple sentences in the vicinity that repeat or reinforce the information.

Air Pollution Harms Your Child's Health

Study results show that air pollution from street traffic gets indoors. The level breathed at home depends on how much traffic is nearby.

Chemicals called PAHs from fuel burning are released into the air in the form of tiny particles and can be harmful to children's health. Remember that air monitor in the backpack you wore before your baby was born? It measured the level of PAHs in air you breathed. Results show that all babies were exposed to PAHs in the womb. As some PAHs are known to cause cancer, this could increase their cancer risk (see how to *Lower Your Child's Cancer Risk* in the box below).

Babies who were exposed in the womb to PAH chemicals *AND* secondhand smoke had worse health than babies who were exposed only to PAHs. Babies exposed to both:

- were born smaller than babies exposed to low levels of both pollutants
- scored lower on tests of learning ability at age two years
- coughed and wheezed more at age one year
- were having more breathing problems and probable asthma diagnoses at two years of age

The map pictured here shows asthma hospitalization rates are highest in areas of Manhattan, where polluting facilities are located close together. Harlem is one of the worst affected neighborhoods in Manhattan, with several bus and garbage truck depots located near each other. Both the

South Bronx and Harlem have some of the highest asthma rates in the country.

Complex Sentences Made Simpler: What the Mothers and Children Study Is Finding Out

Problem: Outdoor air gets inside. When we put a pollution-measuring machine in some of your homes, we found that there was nearly the same amount of black carbon inside your home as outside your home. This means that you and your children are breathing pollution from bus and truck traffic when you are indoors.

Problem: Pollution comes from inside your home too. The machines also measured tiny particles that come from sources inside your home. We found more tiny particles called PAHs indoors than outdoors. This means that pollution is coming from inside homes as well.

What Are PAHs?

PAHs are tiny particles of pollution that get into the air when fuel is burned. They can be very dangerous to children's health.

Where PAHs Come From

- Cars, trucks, buses
- Factories, industry
- Home heating
- Tobacco smoke
- Burned or blackened food
- Burning candles, incense

How You Helped Us Measure the PAHs

When you were pregnant, we gave you a backpack to wear with an air monitor inside. It measured the level of PAHs in the air you breathed. After your baby was born, small samples of blood from you and your baby's umbilical cord also showed how much PAHs from the air were in your bodies.

Source: used by permission from Columbia Center for Children's Environmental Health, *Healthy Home, Healthy Child*, Spring 2005 newsletter, "Air Pollution in Your Neighborhood: What's Being Done to Improve It."

- Vary sentence length.
- Use a complex sentence only when there are simple sentences in the vicinity that repeat or reinforce the information (Exhibit 14.7).
- Use active verbs and sentences. Avoid passive verbs (for example, instead of using "was chosen by the patient," substitute "the patient chose. . . ."). Passives make it hard for the reader to know who did what to whom (Exhibit 14.8).
- Personalize (for example, by using *you* and *we*), but avoid fictitious, hypothetical characters. (Characters will play a role in established narratives or stories and are sometimes necessary to protect confidentiality.)
- Use a good variety of sentence structures. Both simple and compound sentences are used.

Exhibit 14.7. Example: Transforming Long, Complex Sentences.

Hard to Read	*Easier to Read*
During the first 12 months of enrollment, hospitalization and surgical procedures associated with a medical condition diagnosed prior to joining [health plan] require a copayment of 25% of covered services, up to a maximum $1,000 out of pocket per person.	Preexisting Condition: If your doctor told you that you have a medical condition before you joined [health plan], this is called a *preexisting condition*. (Pre Egg ZIS ding).
	If you have to stay at the hospital or have surgery for your preexisting conditions in the first 12 months of your new health plan, then you must pay a copayment. The copayment is what you pay. The copayment will be 25 percent of the covered services, but you will not have to pay more than $1,000 out of pocket.

Exhibit 14.8. Example: Active Versus Passive Form.

Passive Form	Active Form
Anthrax is not known to spread from one person to another.	Scientists (or "we") do not know if anthrax spreads from one person to another.
The evacuation of the area by many people is expected.	We expect many people to evacuate the area.
This is your official notice. You need to choose a health plan by . . . , or a *plan will be chosen for you*. It is best if you make the choice for your family. A plan will be chosen for you.	This is your official notice. You need to choose a health plan by. . . . If you do not choose a health plan by this time, Medicaid will choose a health plan for you.

- Use metaphors and analogies that are meaningful to the audience.
- Use nominal forms sparingly because they are hard to comprehend. Nominals are verbs that work like nouns (see Exhibit 14.9).
- Avoid multiply embedded, packed sentences, for example, "The rat who the dog wearing the red collar chased had just finished eating the cheese." Such a sentence should be broken in two: "A rat ate some cheese and then a dog started to chase it. The dog was wearing a red collar."

Exhibit 14.10 provides a number of examples of difficult sentences and clearer counterparts, and Exhibit 14.11 contains a checklist for writing clear sentences.

Exhibit 14.9. Example: Reducing Use of Nominal Forms.

The evacuation of the area by many people is expected.	We expect many people to evacuate the area.

Exhibit 14.10. Example: Avoiding Multiply Embedded, Packed Sentences.

Hard to Read	Easier to Read
The most common and inexpensive colorectal cancer screening device, FOBT, has an important role in colorectal cancer screening. This test, which can be performed at home and mailed to the medical lab, involves examining a small sample of stool to see if any hidden blood, which you would not be able to see, is present [American College of Gastroenterology, 2005].	FOBT is the most common and least expensive test for colorectal cancer. You can do this test in your own home, and then you can mail it to the medical lab. The test examines a small sample of stool (bowel movement) to see if any hidden blood (blood you cannot see) is there.
Your Medicaid benefits will be discontinued effective 01–31–01 due to the following reasons(s): Failure to cooperate in verifying income. Important: If you believe you may be eligible for Medicaid benefits under another category and have more information about your case, contact your caseworker within 10 days (13 days if this notice is received by mail) of the date of this notice.	Your Medicaid benefits will stop on Jan. 31, 2001. The benefits will stop because: You did not give us the information we asked for. If you have more information about your case and you think you may be eligible for Medicaid, please contact your caseworker in the next 10 days. (If you receive this notice in the mail you have 13 days from the date on the top of this page.) [Zarcadoolas et al., 2001, pp. 15–16].
Public health officials have concluded that secondhand smoke from cigarettes causes disease, including lung cancer and heart disease, in non-smoking adults, as well as causes conditions in children such as	Public health officials know that secondhand smoke from cigarettes cases lung cancer and heart disease in adults even if they do not smoke. Secondhand smoke can cause asthma in

Hard to Read	Easier to Read
asthma, respiratory infections, cough, wheeze, otitis media (middle ear infection) and Sudden Infant Death Syndrome. In addition, public health officials have concluded that second-hand smoke can exacerbate adult asthma and cause eye, throat and nasal irritation [Philip Morris USA, n.d., para. 2].	adults to become worse and they can have eye, throat, and nose irritation. Secondhand smoke can also make children sick. Children can suffer from: • Asthma • Respiratory infections • Cough and wheeze • Ear infections (otitis media) • Sudden infant death syndrome

Exhibit 14.11. Checklist for Writing Clear Sentences.

_____ The sentences are a comfortable length—no more than 7 to 11 words.

_____ The long sentences are simple in structure.

_____ Long sentences have been unpacked into simpler ones.

_____ The sentences are connected smoothly.

_____ The sentences use active voice and avoid passive voice.

_____ The main nouns and verbs are close to each other rather than interrupted by phrases and clauses.

Guideline 4: Text Structure

• Make the most important messages clear, and limit the number of key messages in any text. This example is very hard to read:

Your benefits will be discontinued effective 01/31/06 due to the following reasons(s): FAILURE TO COOPERATE IN VERIFYING INCOME SUPPORTING LAW (S) OR REGULATIONS (S):

The resources, income, and/or expenses of the following individuals were considered in determining your eligibility:
[list names].

Important: If you believe you may be eligible for benefits under another category and have more information about your case, contact your caseworker within 10 days of the date of this notice. The general categories of the Medicaid program are listed below. In addition to meeting the categorical requirements, an individual must also meet specific income and resource requirements which vary according to the category: [list of 16 Medicaid categories].

In the following easier-to-read example, the most important message (MIM) is at the beginning, and the number of messages is limited:

This letter is about your Medicaid benefits. Your benefits will end on January 31, 2006, because you did not give us the information about your income that we asked for.

You may be able to get Medicaid for another reason. To find out, call [name and number of caseworker] by [insert date].

If you get other health insurance you may need proof that you got Medicaid. If you need proof, call your caseworker [name and number same as above] and say, "I'm getting other health insurance and I need proof that I was on Medicaid."

- Use good cohesion.

Cohesion is the glue that holds sentences, paragraphs, and spoken and written text together. Readers and listeners rely on cohesion of all types. The easier-to-read example in Exhibit 14.12 also uses a short narrative (story) structure, which helps the reader or listener.

- Use advance organizers. They signal to the reader, "Get ready to read about . . ." (Exhibit 14.13).
- Use narrative or story structure when appropriate. Using fictional characterization and storytelling (such as in novellas) is help-

Exhibit 14.12. Example: Cohesion.

Hard to Read: Lacks Cohesion	Easier to Read: Has Good Cohesion
Brownfields are abandoned places. Factories used to be in these places. The factories are gone. Sometimes bad chemicals are left behind. These places can be unsafe for people.	Empty or abandoned places are called "brownfields." Factories used to be in these places, but now the factories are gone. When the factories closed down, sometimes they left chemicals in the ground. These chemicals can be danger- ous, and brownfields can be unsafe.

Exhibit 14.13. Example: Advance Organizer.

No Advance Organizer	With Advance Organizer
Most people who get Medicaid must choose a Medicaid health plan for each family member. You get all your Medicaid services from the health plan you choose. You will need to choose a Medic- aid health plan. If you do not choose, we will choose for you!	This letter is about your Medicaid benefits. We want you to know that most people who get Medicaid must choose a Medicaid health plan for each family member.

ful at times, but do not assume that narratives will be appropriate without field testing. Some audiences may find them confusing and irrelevant.

Often message complexity happens on many levels simultane- ously: vocabulary, sentences, and structure—for example:

Protected health information (PHI) is individually identifiable health information, including demographic information collected from you or created or received by a heath care provider, a health plan, your employer, or a health care clearinghouse, and that relates to: (i) your past, present, or future physical or mental health or condition; (ii) the provision of health care to you; or (iii) the past, present or future payment for the provision of health care to you. . . [Blue Cross/Blue Shield of Rhode Island, n.d., p. 1].

In such cases, it is important to systematically use best practice guidelines for written language as well as the other domains of health literacy. Exhibit 14.14 presents a checklist for text structure.

Guideline 5: Giving Instructions

Invariably there is a prescriptive function to most health communication. This often comes in the form of directions or instructions or best practices for the patient or the public. When the situation is charged, as during a natural disaster or other public health emergency, the listener may be more motivated, but the directions must be clear, understandable, and trustworthy:

• Use "in-place" or "just in time" instructions. This means that the instructions appear where or when the consumer or patient is going to need to use them.

Exhibit 14.14. Checklist for General Text Structure.

_____ The most important message appears at the start.

_____ The most important message is repeated.

_____ Advance organizers signal to the reader or listener to get ready to hear about the message.

_____ Good cohesive ties are used within and across sentences and paragraphs.

_____ Instructions are clear, understandable, and in the right place.

- Repeat instructions. This can be especially important in constructing surveys, questionnaires, and forms.
- In spoken language, check to see if the listener can restate the instruction in his or her own words.

Consider this example from a form to be filled out:

What you need to do:

- Be sure to include all the information the form asks for so that we will know if we can meet your needs quickly. We will keep the information you give us confidential (private).
- **Fill out and return** the form in the envelope sent with this letter. **You do not need a stamp**.

Thank you.

These instructions are clear for a number of reasons:

- Bold type highlights key phrases.
- A subhead (advance organizer) tells the reader what type of information is coming next.
- There are no packed complex sentences or passive verb forms.
- The important information is in a list.

Guideline 6: Field Testing

As Yogi Berra has noted, "You observe a lot by watching" (Kaplan, 2001). We recommend field-testing communication approaches and specific messages and texts—in the early stages, in process, and for final evaluation. We conduct field testing to learn about real consumers and patients and to learn about people's awareness, attitudes, perceptions, and understanding of concepts and information.

Qualitative research methods are exploratory and help us refine assumptions about individuals and groups. Ideally, qualitative and quantitative methods should support each other (Ragin, 1994; Ulin, Robinson, & Tolley, 2005).

Collaborating directly with the target audience to conceive, design, and write or script health messages and campaigns is a preferred method for creating campaigns. Models of participatory action research are recommended for ongoing, collaborative exploration (Gaventa, 1993; Park, 1993; Zarcadoolas et al., 2001). These models bring people into the process at the start of a project's design and do not privilege expert knowledge in deciding what is appropriate or most useful. The case studies in Chapters 7 to 13 present important examples of collaborative approaches.

Ethnographic Observation

Ethnographic (participatory) observations are important complements to both one-on-one interviews and focus groups (Gumperz & Hymes, 1964; LeCompte & Schensul, 1999a, 1999b; Fetterman, 1989). Because there are major differences between what people say and what they do, direct observation of one user at a time should be done to supplement focus groups before you make revisions based on focus group data. Observing the way a person uses a tool (an application, handbook, or web site, for example) can help the researcher identify problems in writing and design even when the participant is not able to articulate those problems.

One-on-One Interviews

One-on-one interviews are the most useful way to assess the reader or listener's language and comprehension abilities with a text. Talking and observing will reveal more about the document than soliciting opinions from a focus group. In a one-on-one interview, the researcher can observe:

- Miscues (when the reader reads the wrong word, for example, *parent* for *patient*)

- Difficult vocabulary and sentence structure

- Problems with navigation and design

- The quality of the translation

Use one-on-one interviews for field-testing the suitability of materials. Asking a reader or listener questions about the various elements of the material and observing the participant will tell you much without the interference of group dynamics found in focus group settings.

Focus Groups

Use focus groups for exploring a range of issues with consumers (Morgan, 1993). They are a good way to explore the various types of health literacy at work in a group setting and can be used for gathering group responses about the utility, overall format, and content of materials. They are an excellent way to identify the language people are actually using as they discuss health issues. Focus groups are less satisfactory for precise work on the readability of material.

Cooperative Composing

Use cooperative composing with the target audience to co-create materials and messages (Zarcadoolas et al., 2001). This method is structured as an ongoing process with a panel of consumers or patients to learn with them what types of information they want, what language is appropriate, along with specifics on style and design. This can be done by convening panels of patients or consumers for ongoing input and collaboration.

Guideline 7: Spoken Language

A fuller discussion of the intricacies of spoken language is beyond the scope of this book. The following points are a starting guide for this vital part of health literacy:

- Many people speak at a higher language level than they can read. This means that low-literate readers often speak and use words and sentence structures that they cannot read with comprehension. It is one of the reasons that low literacy is often undetected in social life.
- Consciously check your style and tone of voice to be sure you are engaging the listeners.
- Capitalize on the spoken language skills of consumers.
- Become familiar with the cultural aspects of spoken language. Because culture can and does influence overall speaking style, be aware of cultural differences in conversation style. As discussed in Chapters 12 and 13, culture should be taken into strong consideration when choosing vocabulary, metaphors, appropriate analogies, contexts, and tone. Among the key discourse types that vary greatly across cultures are

Initiating conversations

Opening or closing conversations

Taking turns during conversations

Interrupting

Using silence

Knowing appropriate topics of conversation

Using humor

Using body language to communicate

Guideline 8: Language Translation

As multiculturalism increasingly expands as a value and reality in the world, the ability to communicate critical information in more than one language is a necessity rather than simply a politically correct notion. This is especially true in health care services, where miscommunication can be costly and tragic. A prime weakness in much translation of health information into different languages is that text is translated literally. Many grammatical problems and a lack of cultural approaches are evident in literal translations.

Pictures, drawings, and translations and adaptations have to consider the cultural differences and appropriateness of speakers of languages other than English. We use Spanish here as an example.

Words and phrases in a language have cultural overlays, and it takes personnel who truly know the language and target audience to get the message right. Here are just a few commonly misused terms in Spanish-language health materials (examples provided by Mercedes S. Blanco in a personal communication, 2005):

- *Application* is often translated as *aplicación*. *Aplicación* means assignment. A better choice is *solicitud*.

- *Qualify* (translated as *calificar*) is a false cognate, or Anglicism. *Calificar* means to grade (as in a paper). A more appropriate choice is *reunir los requisitos*.

- The word for Pap smear is *papanicolau* in some Spanish-speaking countries, while in others (Colombia, for example) people talk about *citología* (Zarcadoolas & Blanco, 2000; Blanco, 2001).

We recommend having writers compose original copy in the needed languages. When original writing is not possible, the translator should be given a clear reading level for a nonliteral translation. We call this an adaptation. However, most often health information is written in English and then translated into other languages. Here are some important points to address in working with translations. The text should:

- Accurately reflect the content of the original.

- Address the culture and experience of the target audience.

- Be written at an appropriate literacy level.

- Be written with proper grammar, spelling, and punctuation.

- Approach health communication with respect for the language and culture of the target audience. This requires an approach to translation that is focused on adapting text to accurately convey meaning and intent rather than on literal (word for word) translation.

In addition, it is important to:

- Rigorously use back translation to check the quality and appropriateness of the text.

- Use pictures, drawings, and translation or adaptations respecting cultural differences and appropriateness of the target audience.

When working with a translator, follow these guidelines:

- Choose a native speaker who writes well in his or her primary language and knows English as well. If translators are proficient in their native language but not in English, they will have trouble understanding the meaning of the original document.

- Do not ask an interpreter to do translations. Interpreters explain or translate orally; translators are trained writers. The ability to translate is a skill quite different from the skills involved in oral language. Just as all speakers of English are not automatically good writers, so too all speakers of other languages are not automatically good translators and writers.

- Choose a translator experienced in writing for low-literate consumers and knowledgeable about health care concepts.

Writing specifically for these consumers is a special skill. The translator has to convey complicated health-related concepts using simple vocabulary and an uncomplicated sentence structure.

- Make sure the translator is familiar with the health care concepts in your material and has translated documents with similar concepts.

- When possible, translators should participate in field testing.

Guideline 9: Web Design

Vast stores of health information are available on the web, but it is often hard to find and read. The following are basic guidelines for web usability. There is growing agreement that much of the internet is poorly designed in terms of the ability to help people with low literacy and health literacy skills. These guidelines are based on our own research and the best practices of others.

- Web pages that are packed with graphics or text present multiple barriers to low-literate readers.
- Graphics should be clearly labeled and functional.
- Active graphics (those that are used as navigation devices) should be accompanied by clear, simple instructions.
- Where possible, designers should not require scrolling or explicitly inform users that more information is below the browser frame.
- Spelling difficulties should be taken into consideration when designing search interfaces. Some search engines now suggest alternate spellings of search words.

- Provide multiple means of entering pages, for example, table of contents, links to the side, links at the bottom, and links at the top.
- Web users, like readers, are not all the same. Therefore, layer the complexity of your site so that basic information can be found easily and users can drill down to more complex information as needed.
- Include instructions to users and helpful tips.
- Displaying a user's path history on each page allows them an easy method to retrace their steps.
- Building a web site that is only in English is roughly analogous to establishing a business in every capital city of the world but hiring only English-speaking employees.

Guideline 10: Graphics and Layout of Print Materials

The major purpose of graphics and layout should be to highlight and reinforce key messages, not to glamorize. In an attempt to be more contemporary, some designers overdesign material: it looks good but defies basic readability elements. Use graphic elements (such as illustrations and photographs) to support the message and create some visual relief from the text. A few well-chosen graphics can greatly increase the friendliness of print material.

The critical role of design is to present messages in a way that people want to read (appeal), can read quickly (accessibility and comprehension), and can remember what they read (reinforcement). Illustrations should enhance and emphasize the message. They should be clear and be appropriate for age, gender, and other sociological contexts of the individuals. School-based elements, such as graphs and charts, should be simplified or not used at all.

Here are some specific points:

- Avoid a wall of print. For easiest reading, sentence length should be 5 to 11 words. Avoid text lines that run the full width of a standard page because a reader's eye can easily get lost. Use narrower columns, and supply ample white space around headlines, graphics, and logos.

- If you are in doubt about layout, use the designers' "Z," reading across, down, and across. The natural movement of the eye is left to right and top to bottom. Use an optical at the bottom left to move the eye to that position after going across the top.
- Do not use overprinting (text printed over visuals).
- Avoid complicated folding.
- Do not unnecessarily interrupt the text with graphic elements such as changes in columns, color, or the flow of text on the page. Interrupted flow is one of the biggest obstacles to readers.
- Choose typefaces that make individual letters easy to distinguish. This often is a serif typeface. Choose one typeface for headlines and subheads and another for the body text. Some clear typefaces are Times New Roman, Garamond, Palatino, and Futura. Do not change typefaces within a run of text.
- Avoid underlining because the bottoms of letters can be cut off.
- Text wrapping around a graphic is okay, but avoid complicated, jagged wraparounds.
- Avoid using all caps; they are hard to read.

Guideline 11: Media

Beyond the fundamental skills of reading, watching, and listening there is a range of conceptual hurdles to becoming a savvy media consumer. We suggest the following are important to adopt in practice as well as teaching and outreach:

- Be aware of the difference between news, opinion, and advertising.

- Pay attention to the different ways of telling stories in each medium. Also understand how each medium offers information in different ways relating to the type of communication involved: print, visual, or verbal.

- Realize there is a difference between the reality presented in the mass media and actual practice in life.

- Be attuned to the differing functions of the media: gatekeeping, surveillance, and framing, for example.

- Consider news coverage as an ongoing narrative rather than a series of snapshots.

- Pay attention to the presentation of uncertainty in science and health coverage.

- Consider the source of the news: all sources are not equal.

- Understand that a media agenda can determine the content of the mass media and the news.

- Consider the distinction between reality as you experience it and reality as presented by the media.

- Look for coverage of the same event or idea in multiple mass media outlets in order to get a broader point of view.

- Physicians and patients should seek information from noncorporate funded sources.

- Government and other noncommercial entities should produce accessible materials on conditions and diseases.

- Widen your notion of informed consent to include information about controversy surrounding the definitions of conditions and diseases.

- Realize that the choice of product and brands in movies and TV shows is likely dictated not by the actor's preference but by a commercial arrangement.

The preceding guidelines are meant as basic signposts for planning and designing health communications. As you become more aware of health literacy issues and the particular needs of your target audience, you will find your own methods to bridge the gap between expert and lay communications.

References

Abt Associates. (2000). *Independent evaluation of the Massachusetts Tobacco Control Program: January 1994 to June 2000* (Tech. Rep. No. 7). Boston: Massachusetts Department of Public Health.

Achard, M., & Kemmer, S. (Eds.). (2004). *Language, culture and mind.* Palo Alto, CA: Center for the Study of Language and Information, Stanford University.

AdAge.com. (2002). *Magazines by circulation for 6 mos. ended 12/31/2002* [Electronic version]. AdAge.com. Retrieved Mar. 1, 2003, from http://www.adage.com/page.cms?pageId=971.

Ad Hoc Committee on Health Literacy for the Council on Scientific Affairs. (1999, Feb. 10). Health literacy: Report of the Council on Scientific Affairs. *Journal of the American Medical Association, 281*(6), 552–557.

Aikin, K. J. (2002). *Direct-to-consumer advertising of prescription drugs: physician survey preliminary results* [Online report]. Division of Drug Marketing, Advertising, and Communications, Center for Drug Evaluation and Research, U.S. Food and Drug Administration. Retrieved Feb. 18, 2004, from www.fda.gov/cder/ddmac/globalsummit2003/.

American Cancer Society. (2006). What are the risk factors for colorectal cancer? (para. 1 & 2). Retrieved Jan. 27, 2006, from http://www.cancer.org/docroot/CRI/content/CRI_2_4_2X_What_are_the_risk_factors_for_colon_and_rectum_cancer.asp?sitearea=CRI.

American College of Gastroenterology. (2005). *Medicare covers a test that could save your life.* Retrieved Sept. 10, 2005, from http://www.acg.gi.org/patients/ccrk/medicare_brochure.asp.

American Diabetes Association. (n.d.). *All about diabetes* [Web site]. Retrieved Feb. 19, 2004, from http://www.diabetes.org/about-diabetes.jsp.

American Evaluation Association. (1994). *Guiding principles for evaluators.* American Evaluation Association Task Force. Retrieved Jan. 10, 2004, from http://www.eval.org/EvaluationDocuments/aeaprin6.html.

American Medical Association Foundation. (2003). *Health literacy: Help your patients understand* [Video]. Chicago: American Medical Association.

Anderson, A. (1997). *Media, culture and the environment.* New Brunswick, NJ: Rutgers University Press.

Andreason, A. R. (1995). *Marketing social change: Changing behavior to promote health, social development, and the environment.* San Francisco: Jossey-Bass.

Aragon, R., Kates, J., Greene, L., & Hoff, T. (2001). *The AIDS epidemic at 20 years: The view from America.* Menlo Park, CA: Henry J. Kaiser Family Foundation.

Atkin, C. (1982). Television advertising and socialization to consumer roles. In D. Pearl, L. Bouthilet, & J. Lazar (Eds.), *Television and behavior: Ten years of scientific progress and implications for the eighties* (pp. 191–200). Rockville, MD: National Institute of Mental Health.

Bailey, M. (1991). Community-based organizations and CDC as partners in HIV education and prevention. *Public Health Reports, 106*(6), 702–708.

Baker, C. (1999). *Your genes, your choices.* Washington, DC: American Association for the Advancement of Science.

Baker, D. W., Williams, M. V., Parker, R. M., Gazmarian, J. A., & Nurss, J. (1999). Development of a brief test to measure functional health literacy. *Patient Education and Counseling, 38,* 33–42.

Baltimore, D. (n.d.). *DNA is reality beyond metaphor* [Web site]. California Institute of Technology. Retrieved Aug. 10, 2003, from http://pr.caltech.edu/events/dna/dnabalt2.html.

Bandura, A., & Cervone, D. (1983). Self-evaluative and self-efficacy mechanisms governing motivational effects of goal systems. *Journal of Personality and Social Psychology, 45,* 1017–1028.

Bell, A. (1991). *The language of the news media.* Cambridge, MA: Blackwell.

Berke, R. L., & Elder, J. (2001). Survey shows doubts stirring on terror war [Electronic version]. *New York Times.* Retrieved Jan. 18, 2001, from http://www.nytimes.com/2001/10/30/national/30POLL.html.

Berkowitz, B. (2000). Collaboration for health improvement: Models for state, community, and academic partnerships. *Journal of Public Health Management and Practice, 6*(1), 67–72.

Berland, G. K., Elliott, M. N., Morales, L. S., Algazy, J. I., Kravitz, R. L., Broder, M. S., Kanouse, D. E., Muoz, J., Puyol, J., Lara, M., Watkins, K. E., Yang, H., & McGlynn, E. A. (2001). Health information on the internet:

Accessibility, quality, and readability in English and Spanish. *Journal of the American Medical Association, 285*(20), 2612–2621.

Bessell, T. L., McDonald, S., Silagy, C. A., Anderson, J. N., Hiller, J. E., & Sansom, L. N. (2002). Do internet interventions for consumers cause more harm than good? A systematic review. *Health Expectations, 5*(1), 28–37.

Bettman, J. R. (1975). Issues in designing consumer information environments. *Journal of Consumer Research, 2*, 169–177.

Biener, L., McCallum-Keeler, G., & Nyman, A. L. (2000). Adults' response to Massachusetts anti-tobacco television advertisements: Impact of viewer and advertisement characteristics. *Tobacco Control, 9*, 401–407.

Binson, D., & Catania, J. A. (1998). Respondents' understanding of the words used in sexual behavior questions. *Public Opinion Quarterly, 62*(2), 190–208.

Blanco, M. (2001, Nov. 1). *Lost in translation.* Presented at the Eligibility Conference, Center for Medicare and Medicaid Services, Atlanta, GA.

Blendon, R. J., Benson, J. M., DesRoches, C. M., & Herrmann, M. J. (2001). *Survey project on Americans' response to biological terrorism.* Media, PA: Harvard School of Public Health/Robert Wood Johnson Foundation.

Blendon, R., Young, J., & DesRoches, C. (1999). The uninsured, the working uninsured, and the public. *Health Affairs, 18*(6), 203–211.

Blue Cross/Blue Shield of Rhode Island. (n.d.) Health Insurance Portability and Accountability Act (HIPAA). *Notice of privacy practices* [Online notice]. Rhode Island Blue Cross/Blue Shield. Retrieved Feb. 17, 2004, from http://www.bcbsri.com/BCBSRIWeb/help/fullyinsured.pdf.

Botta, R. A. (1999). Television images and adolescent girls' body image disturbance. *Journal of Communication, 49*(2), 22–41.

Bransford, J. D., & Johnson, M. K. (1972). Contextual prerequisites for understanding: Some investigations of comprehension and recall. *Journal of Verbal Learning and Verbal Behavior, 11*(6), 717–726.

Britton, B., & Graesser, A. (1996). *Models of understanding text.* Mahwah, NJ: Erlbaum.

Brown, P., & Mikkelsen, E. J. (1997). *No safe place.* Berkeley: University of California Press.

Bruner, J. S. (1966). *Toward a theory of instruction.* Cambridge, MA: Harvard University Press.

Bryman, A. (1992). *Quantity and quality in social research.* London: Routledge.

Burton, B. (2003). Ban direct to consumer advertising, report recommends. *BMJ, 326*(7387), 467.

Campaign for Tobacco-Free Kids. (2003). *Summary of the Multistate Settlement Agreement (MSA)*. National Center for Tobacco-Free Kids. Retrieved Mar. 15, 2004, from http://www.tobaccofreekids.org.

Campaign for Tobacco-Free Kids, American Lung Association, American Cancer Association, American Heart Association, & SmokeLess States National Tobacco Policy Initiative. (2003). *Show us the money: A report on the states' allocation of the tobacco settlement dollars:* Campaign for Tobacco-Free Kids. Retrieved Mar. 15, 2004, from http://www.tobaccofreekids.org.

Cancela, D. L., Chim, J. L., & Jenkins, Y. M. (1998). *Community health psychology: Empowerment for diverse communities*. New York: Routledge.

Cannon, A. (2001, Nov. 5). Unlikely foot soldiers in the war against terror. *U.S. News and World Report, 18*.

Cargo, M., Lévesque, L., Macaulay, A. C., McComber, A., Desrosiers, S., Delormier, T., & Potvin, L. (2003). Community governance of the Kahnawake Schools Diabetes Prevention Project, Kahnawake Territory, Mohawk Nation, Canada. *Health Promotion International, 18*(3), 177–187.

Carmines, E. G., & Zeller, R. A. (1979). *Reliability and validity assessment*. Thousand Oaks, CA: Sage.

Carrigan, J. A. (1994). *The saffron scourge: A history of yellow fever in Louisiana, 1796–1905*. Lafayette: Center for Louisiana Studies, University of Southwestern Louisiana.

Casey, M., Allen, M., Emmers-Sommer, T., Sahlstein, E., Degooyer, D., Winters, A. M., Wagner, A. E., & Dun, T. (2003). When a celebrity contracts a disease: The example of Earvin Magic Johnson's announcement that he was HIV positive. *Journal of Health Communication, 8*(3), 249–265.

Centers for Disease Control and Prevention. (1998a). *HIV prevention community planning: Shared decision making in action*. Retrieved Nov. 21, 2002, from http://cdc.gov/hiv/pubs/guidelines.htm.

Centers for Disease Control and Prevention. (1998b). Incidence of initiation of cigarette smoking: United States, 1965–1996. *Morbidity and Mortality Weekly Report, 47*(39), 837–840.

Centers for Disease Control and Prevention. (1999). *1999 Healthstyles survey: Soap opera viewers and health information*. Retrieved Mar. 1, 2003, from http://www.cdc.gov/communication/healthsoap.htm#findings.

Centers for Disease Control and Prevention. (2001). *HIV prevention strategic plan through 2005*. Atlanta, GA: Author. Retrieved Nov. 21, 2002, from http://cdc.gov/nchstp/od/news/prevention.pdf.

Centers for Disease Control and Prevention. (2002a). Cigarette smoking among adults: United States, 2000. *Morbidity and Mortality Weekly Report, 51*(29), 642–645.

Centers for Disease Control and Prevention. (2002b). *Definition.* Center for Disease Control, Atlanta. Retrieved Sept. 29, 2002 from http://www.bt.cdc.gov/agent/faq/definition.asp.

Centers for Disease Control and Prevention. (2003). *Tobacco information and prevention source* [Web site]. Office of Smoking and Health. Retrieved Sept. 9, 2003, from http://www.cdc.gov/tobacco.

Centers for Disease Control and Prevention. (2004). *Colorectal cancer: The importance of prevention and early detection* [Electronic version]. Atlanta, GA: Author. Retrieved Sept. 1, 2005, from http://www.cdc.gov/cancer/colorctl/about2004.htm.

Centers for Disease Control and Prevention. (2006, Feb. 7). Key facts about avian influenza (bird flu) and avian influenza A (H5N1) virus. Retrieved Jan. 28, 2006, from http://www.cdc.gov/flu/avian/gen-info/facts.htm.

Chadwick, H. D., & Pope, A. S. (1946). *The modern attack on tuberculosis.* New York: Commonwealth Fund.

Chang, J., Elam-Evans, L. D., Berg, C. J., Herndon, J., Flowers, L., Seed, K. A., & Syverson, C. J. (2003, Feb. 21). Pregnancy-related mortality surveillance: United States, 1991–1999. *Morbidity and Mortality Weekly Report,* 1–8.

Clanchy, M. T. (1979). *From memory to written record: England, 1066–1307.* London: Edward Arnold.

Clenland, J. G., & Van Ginniken, J. K. (1988). Maternal education and child survival in developing countries: The search for pathways of influence. *Social Science Medicine, 27*(1), 357–368.

Cohen, L. H., Fine, B. A., & Pergament, E. (1998). An assessment of ethnocultural beliefs regarding the causes of birth defects and genetic disorders. *Journal of Genetic Counseling, 7*(1), 15–19.

Cohn, V. (1955, Apr.). *Four billion dimes.* Minneapolis, MN: Minneapolis Star and Tribune.

Coleman, J. (1990). *Foundations of social theory.* Cambridge, MA: Harvard University Press.

Collier, P. (1998). *Social capital and poverty.* Washington, DC: World Bank.

Collins, F. S., & Bochm, K. (1999). Avoiding casualties in the genetic revolution: The urgent need to educate physicians about genetics. *Academic Medicine, 74*(1), 48–49.

Collins, F. S., & Guttmacher, A. E. (2001). Genetics moves into the medical mainstream. JAMA, 286(18), 2322–2324.

Commission on Macroeconomics and Health. (2001). *Macroeconomics and health: Investing in health for economic development* [Electronic version]. Retrieved Sept. 1, 2005, from http://www.cmhealth.org.

Committee on Communications. (1995). Children, adolescents, and advertising. *Pediatrics, 95*(2), 295–297.

Committee on Public Education. (1999). Media education. *Pediatrics, 104*(2), 341–343.

Committee on Public Education. (2001). Children, adolescents, and television. *Pediatrics, 107*(2), 423–426.

Concato, J., Shah, N., & Horwitz, R. I. (2000). Randomized, controlled trials, observational studies, and the hierarchy of research designs. *New England Journal of Medicine, 342*(25), 1887–1892.

Condit, C. M. (1999). *The meanings of the gene: Public debates about human heredity*. Madison: University of Wisconsin Press.

Connolly, C. (2001, Nov. 8). U.S. officials reorganize strategy on bioterrorism. *Washington Post,* A1.

Cottrell, L. (1977). The competent community. In R. Warren (Ed.), *New perspectives on the American community* (pp. 535–545). Skokie, IL: Rand McNally.

Curran, J. (2002, Sept. 19). Remarks presented at Fifth Annual Pfizer Health Literacy Conference, Washington, DC.

David, S. P., & Greer, D. S. (2001). Social marketing: Application to medical education. *Annals of Internal Medicine, 134*(2), 125–127.

Davis, M. (2003). *Discussion of reading memes*. Retrieved Feb. 9, 2004, from http://www.mrc-cbu.cam.ac.uk/~mattd/Cmabrigde/index.html.

Davis, T., Crouch, M., Wills, G., Miller, S., & Abdehou, D. (1990). Gap between patient reading comprehension and the readability of patient education materials. *Journal of Family Practice, 31*(5), 533–538.

DeFleur, M. L., & Dennis, E. E. (2002). *Understanding mass communication: A liberal arts perspective*. Boston: Houghton Mifflin.

Dela, C., Chim, J. L., & Jenkins, Y. M. (1998). *Community health psychology: Empowerment for diverse communities*. New York: Routledge.

Dickson, D. A., Hargie, O., & Morrow, N. C. (1989). *Communication skills training for health professionals—An instructor handbook*. London: Chapman and Hall.

Dierkes, M., & von Grote, C. (Eds.). (2000). *Between understanding and trust: The public, science and technology*. Amsterdam: Harwood Academic Publishers.

Digital Divide Network. (2005). *Empowering those displaced by the hurricane*. Retrieved Sept. 10, 2005, from http:///www.digitaldivide.net.

Dijk, J. V. (1998). *Imagenation: Popular images of genetics*. New York: New York University Press.

DiversityRX. (2005). *Why language and culture are important*. Retrieved July 6, 2005, from http://www.diversityrx.org/HTML/ESLANG.htm.

Division of Reproductive Health. (n.d.). *Reproductive health: Home*. Centers for Disease Control. Retrieved Sept. 1, 2005, from www.cdc.gov/reproductivehealth/index.htm.

DNA Files. (1998). *Predictive genetic tests: Do you really want to know your future?* [Electronic version]. Retrieved Sept. 1, 2005, from http://www.dnafiles.org/.

Doak, C. C., Doak, L. G., & Root, J. (1996). *Teaching patients with low literacy skills*. Philadelphia: Lippincott.

Doak, L. G., & Doak, C. C. (2002). *Pfizer health literacy principles*. New York: Pfizer (produced by SoundVision® Productions).

Dolan DNA Learning Center. (2003). *Image archive on the American eugenics movement* [Web site]. Cold Spring Harbor Laboratory. Retrieved Sept. 3, 2003, from http://www.eugenicsarchive.org.

Donovan, K. A., & Tucker, D. C. (2000). Knowledge about genetic risk for breast cancer and perceptions of genetic testing in a sociodemographically diverse sample. *Journal of Behavioral Medicine, 23*(1), 15–36.

Eisenberg, A., Murkoff, H., & Hathaway, S. E.. (2002). *What to expect when you're expecting* (3rd ed.). New York: Workman.

Emery, J., Watson, E., Rose, P., & Andermann, A. (1999). A systematic review of the literature exploring the role of primary care in genetic services. *Family Practice, 6*(4), 425–445.

Environmental Protection Agency. (1999). *Consumer labeling initiative*. Retrieved Sept. 1, 2005, from http://www.epa.gov/opptintr/labeling/.

Epstein, S. (1995). The construction of lay expertise: AIDS activism and the forging of credibility in the reform of clinical trials. *Science, Technology and Human Values, 20*(4), 408–437.

Epstein, S. (2000). Democracy, expertise, and AIDS treatment activism. In D. Kleinman (Ed.), *Science, technology and democracy* (pp. 15–32). Albany: State University of New York Press.

Erzinger, S. (1991). Communication between Spanish-speaking patients and their doctors in medical encounters. *Culture, Medicine and Psychiatry, 15*, 91–110.

Evans, S. H., & Clarke, P. (1983). When cancer patients fail to get well: Flaws in health communication. In R. Bostrom (Ed.), *Communication Yearbook 7*. Thousand Oaks, CA: Sage.

Eysenbach, G. (2000). Toward ethical guidelines for e-health: JMIR theme issue on eHealth ethics. *Journal of Medical Internet Research, 2*(1), e7.

Eysenbach, G., & Kohler, C., (2004). Health-related searches on the internet. *JAMA, 291*(24), 2946.

Eysenbach G., Sa, E. R., & Diepgen, T. L. (1999). Shopping around the internet today and tomorrow: Towards the millennium of cybermedicine. *BMJ, 319*(7220), 1294.

Fadiman, A. (1997). *The spirit catches you and you fall down: A Hmong child, her American doctors, and the collision of two cultures*. New York: Farrar, Straus, and Giroux.

Fetterman, D. M. (1989). *Ethnography step by step*. Thousand Oaks, CA: Sage.

Fillmore, C. (1974). Pragmatics and the description of discourse. In C. Fillmore, G. Lakoff, & R. Lakoff (Eds.), *Berkeley studies in syntax and semantics*. Berkeley: Institute of Human Learning, Department of Linguistics, University of California.

Findlay, S. D. (2001). Direct-to-consumer promotion of prescription drugs: Economic implications for patients, payers and providers. *Pharmacoeconomics, 19*(2), 109–119.

Fingeret, H. A. (1990). Changing literacy instruction: Moving beyond the status quo. In F. P. Chisman & Associates, *Leadership for literacy: The agenda for the 1990s*. San Francisco: Jossey-Bass. (ED 323 819)

Fingeret, H. A. (1992). *Adult literacy education: Current and future directions. An update* (Information Series No. 355). Columbus, OH: ERIC Clearinghouse on Adult, Career, and Vocational Education, Center on Education for Training and Employment. (ED 354 391)

Fischhoff, B. (1989). Making decisions about AIDS. In S. Schneider (Ed.), *Primary prevention of AIDS*. Thousand Oaks, CA: Sage.

Flores, G., Abreu, M., Olivar, M. A., & Kastner, B. (1998). Access barriers to health care for Latino children. *Archives of Pediatric and Adolescent Medicine, 152*, 1119–1125.

Fogle, T. (1995). Information metaphors and the human genome project. *Perspectives in Biology and Medicine, 38*(4), 535–547.

Fox, S., & Rainie, L. (2000). *The on-line health care revolution: How the web helps Americans take better care of themselves*. Retrieved Sept. 21, 2002, from http://www.pewinternet.org/reports/toc.asp?Report=26.

Frank, R. G., Berndt, E. R., Donahue, J. M., Epstein, A. M., & Rosenthal, M. B. (2002). *Trends in direct-to-consumer advertising of prescription drugs*. Menlo Park, CA: Kaiser Family Foundation.

Friedman, S. M., Dunwoody, S., & Rogers, C. L. (Eds.). (1999). *Communicating uncertainty: Media coverage of new and controversial science*. Mahwah, NJ: Erlbaum.

Gaither, C., & Gold, M. (2005, Sept. 10). Web proves its capacity to help in time of need. *Los Angeles Times*. Retrieved Apr. 3, 2006, from http://mediachannel.org/blog/node/959.

Gannett Corporation. (2002). *Company profile*. Retrieved May 1, 2002, from http://www.gannett.com/map/gan007.htm.

Gaventa, J. (1993). The powerful, the powerless, and the experts: Knowledge struggles in the information age. In P. Park, J. Gaventa, T. Heaney, T. Jackson, J. Merrifield, B. D. Horton, D. E. Comstock, R. Fox, M. Brydon-Miller, M. B. Castellano, & P. Maguire (Eds.), *Voices of change: Participatory research in the United States and Canada* (pp. 20–40). Westport, CT: Bergin & Garvey.

Gazmararian, J. A. (1999). Health literacy among Medicare enrollees in a managed care organization. *Journal of the American Medical Association, 281*, 545–551.

General Social Survey. (2000). Retrieved Sept. 1, 2005, from http://www.cpanda.org/data/a00032/a00032.html.

Gibbs, R. W., Jr. (1996). Metaphor as a constraint on text understanding. In B. K. Britton & A. C. Graesser (Eds.), *Models of understanding text* (pp. 215–240). Mahwah, NJ: Erlbaum.

Gigerenzer, G., & Edwards, A. (2003). Simple tools for understanding risks: From innumeracy to insight. *BMJ, 327*(7417), 741–744.

Giovino, G. A. (2002). Epidemiology of tobacco use in the United States. *Oncogene, 21*(48), 7326–7340.

Gittell, R., & Vidal, A. (1997). *Community organizing*. Thousand Oaks, CA: Sage.

Glanz, K., & Rudd, J. (1990). Readability and content analysis of print cholesterol education materials. *Patient Education and Counseling, 16*(2), 109–117.

Glucksberg, S. (1989). Metaphors in conversation: How are they understood? Why are they used? *Metaphor and Symbolic Activity, 4*, 125–144.

Goffman, E. (1981). *Forms of talk*. Philadelphia: University of Pennsylvania Press.

Gohdes, D. (1988). Diet therapy for minority patients with diabetes. *Diabetes Care, 11*(2), 189–191.

Gohdes, D. (1995). Diabetes in North American Indians and Alaska Natives. In M. I. Harris, C. C. Cowie, M. P. Stern, E. J. Boyko, G. E. Reiber, and P. H. Bennett (Eds.), *Diabetes in America* (2nd ed., pp. 683–701). Bethesda, MD: National Institute of Diabetes and Digestive and Kidney Diseases, National Institutes of Health.

Goldman, L. K., & Glantz, S. A. (1998). Evaluation of antismoking advertising campaigns. *Journal of the American Medical Association, 279*(10), 772–777.

Gollust, S. E., Hull, S. C., & Wilfond, B. S. (2002). Limitations of direct-to-consumer advertising for clinical genetic testing. *Journal of the American Medical Association, 288*(14), 1762–1767.

Goody, J., & Watt, I. (1968). The consequences of literacy. In J. Goody (Ed.), *Literacy in traditional societies*. Cambridge, England: Cambridge University Press.

Gottlieb, S. (2002). A fifth of Americans contact their doctor as a result of drug advertising. *BMJ, 325*(7369), 854.

Graber, M. A., Roller, C. M., & Kaeble, B. (1999). Readability levels of patient education material on the World Wide Web. *Journal of Family Practice, 48*(1), 58–61.

Green, S. K., Lightfoot, M. A., Bandy, C., & Buchanan, D. R. (1985). A general model of the attribution process. *Basic and Applied Social Psychology, 6*(2), 159–179.

Greenfield, P. M. (1972). Oral or written language: The consequences for cognitive development in Africa, the United States, and England. *Language and Speech, 15*(2), 169–178.

Gregory, J., & Miller, S. (1998). *Science in public: Communication, culture, and credibility*. Cambridge, MA: Perseus Publishing.

Griffiths, W. (1972). Health education definitions, problems, and philosophies. *Health Education Monographs, 31*, 12–14.

Grosse, R. N., & Auffrey, B. (1989). Literacy and health status in developing countries. *Annual Review of Public Health, 10*, 281–297.

Gumperz, J. J. (Ed.). (1982). *Language and social identity*. Cambridge, England: Cambridge University Press.

Gumperz, J. J., & Hymes, D. (Eds.). (1964). *Ethnography of communication*. Menasha, WI: American Anthropological Association.

Gunn, S. M., & Platt, P. S. (1945). *Voluntary health agencies: An interpretive study*. New York: Ronald Press.

Haas, S., & Grams, E. (2000). Readers, authors and page structure: A discussion of four questions arising from content analysis of web pages. *Journal of the American Society for Information Science, 51*(2), 181–192.

Hall, S. (1996). Gramsci's relevance for the study of race and ethnicity. In D. Morley & K. Chew (Eds.), *Stuart Hall: Critical dialogues in cultural studies* (pp. 411–440). New York: Routledge.

Halliday, M.A.K., & Hasan, R. (1976). *Cohesion in English*. White Plains, NY: Longman.

Harris Interactive. (2001). Retrieved Feb. 24, 2004, from http://www.harrisinteractive.com/harris_poll.

Harrison, K., & Cantor, J. (1997). The relationship between media consumption and eating disorders. *Journal of Communication, 47*(1), 40–68.

Havelock, E. A. (1973). Prologue to Greek literacy. In E. Sjóqvist (Ed.), *Lectures in memory of Louise Taft Semple* (pp. 329–391). Cincinnati, OH: University of Oklahoma Press for the University of Cincinnati.

Health Care Financing Administration. (1998). *Medicaid managed care state enrollment—December 31, 1998*. Baltimore: MD: Author. Retrieved Aug. 10, 2004, from www.hcfa.gov/medicaid/omcpr98.htm.

Hohn, M. D. (1997). *Empowerment health education in adult literacy: A guide for public health and adult literacy practitioners, policy makers and funders* [Online report]. National Institute for Literacy. Retrieved Feb. 15, 2004, from http://www.nifl.gov/nifl/fellowship/reports/hohn/HOHN.HTM.

Holahan, J., & Brennan, N. (2000). *Who are the adult uninsured?* Washington, DC: Urban Institute.

Hollon, M. F. (2005). Direct-to-consumer advertising: A haphazard approach to health promotion. *Journal of the American Medical Association, 293,* 2030–2033.

Hubbard, R., & Wald, E. (1993). *Exploding the gene myth: How genetic information is produced and manipulated by scientists, physicians, employers, insurance companies, educators, and law enforcers*. Boston: Beacon Press.

Hymes, D. (1974). *Foundations of sociolinguistics: An ethnographic approach*. Philadelphia: University of Pennsylvania Press.

Institute for the Future. (2003). *Health and health care 2010: The forecast, the challenge* (2nd ed.). San Francisco: Jossey-Bass.

Institute for the Future. (2004, Jan.). *Expanded meanings of health* (Report SR-815B). Menlo Park, CA: Author. Retrieved Feb. 7, 2006, from http://www.iftf.org/docs/SR-815B_Meanings_of_Health.pdf.

Institute of Medicine. (1988). *The future of public health*. Washington, DC: National Academy Press.

Institute of Medicine. (2003). *The future of the public's health in the 21st century*. Washington, DC: National Academy Press.

International Adult Literacy Survey. (2003). *Reading the future: A portrait of literacy in Canada—Highlights from the Canadian report* [Web site]. Human Resources Development Canada. Retrieved Sept. 1, 2005, from http://www.hrsdc.gc.ca/en/hip/lld/nls/Surveys/ialscrh.shtml.

Jacobs, P. P. (1940). *The control of tuberculosis in the United States*. New York: National Tuberculosis Association.

Jacoby, J. (1977). Consumer use and comprehension of nutrition information. *Journal of Consumer Research, 4*, 119–128.

Jakobsen, R. (1978). Closing statement: Linguistics and poetics. In T. A. Sebeok (Ed.), *Style in language* (pp. 350–377). Cambridge, MA: MIT Press.

Jallinoja, P., & Aro, A. R. (2000). Does knowledge make a difference? The association between knowledge about genes and attitudes toward gene tests. *Journal of Health Communication, 5*, 29–39.

Jamieson, K. H., & Campbell, K. K. (1997). *Interplay of influence: News, advertising, politics, and the mass media* (4th ed.). Belmont, CA: Wadsworth.

Janssen, W. F. (1981). Outline of the history of U. S. drug regulation and labeling. *Food, Drug, Cosmetic Law Journal, 36*, 420-441.

Jaroff, L. (1989, Mar. 20). The gene hunt. *Time*, p. 67.

Jasanoff, S. (1997). Civilization and madness: The great BSE scare of 1996. *Public Understanding of Science, 6*(3), 221–232.

Jolly, B. T., Scott, J., Feied, C. F., & Sanford, S. M. (1993). Functional illiteracy among emergency department patients: A preliminary study. *Annals of Emergency Medicine, 22*(3), 573–578.

Jones, J. M. (2001). *Concern about anthrax exposure remains low* [Electronic version]. Princeton, NJ: Gallup Organization. Retrieved Jan. 25, 2002, from http://www.gallup.com.

Kaphingst, K. A., Rudd, R. E., DeJong, W., & Daltroy, L. (2004a). A content analysis of direct-to-consumer television prescription drug advertisements. *Journal of Health Communication, 9*(6), 515–528.

Kaphingst, K. A., Rudd, R. E., DeJong, W., & Daltroy, L. (2004b). Literacy demands of product information intended to supplement television direct-to-consumer prescription drug advertisements. *Patient Education Counseling, 55*(2), 293–300.

Kaplan, D. (2001). *When you come to a fork in the road, take it!* New York: Hyperion.

Kawachi, I., & Berkman, L. F. (1998). Social cohesion, social capital and health. In L. F. Berkman & I. Kawachi (Eds.), *Social epidemiology*. New York: Oxford University Press.

Kawachi, I., Kennedy, B. P., & Prothrow-Stith, D. (1997). Social capital, income inequality, and mortality. *American Journal of Public Health, 87,* 1491–1498.

Kerka, S. (2003). *Health literacy beyond basic skills* [Electronic version]. Washington, DC: U.S. Department of Education, Educational Resources Information Center; 2003 (ERIC digest; no. 245;). Retrieved Sept. 10, 2005, from http://www.cete.org/acve/docs/dig245.pdf.

Kickbusch, I. (1997). Think health: What makes the difference. *Health Promotion International, 12*(4), 265–272.

Kickbusch, I. (2001). Health literacy: Addressing the health and education divide. *Health Promotion International, 16*(3), 289–297.

Kintsch, W. (1977). On comprehending stories. In M. A. Just & P. A. Carpenter (Eds.), *Cognitive processes in comprehension* (pp. 33–61). Mahwah, NJ: Erlbaum.

Kintsch, W., Kozminsky, E., Streby, W. J., McKoon, G., & Keenan, J. M. (1975). Comprehension and recall of text as a function of content variables. *Journal of Verbal Learning and Verbal Behavior, 14,* 196–214.

Kirsch, J. S., Junegeblut, A., Jenkins, L., & Kolstad, L. A. (1993). *Adult literacy in America: A first look at the results of the National Adult Literacy Survey (NALS).* Washington, DC: Department of Education.

Klare, G. R. (1963). *The measurement of readability.* Iowa City: Iowa University Press.

Knapp, M. L., & Hall, J. A. (2002). *Nonverbal communication in human interaction* (5th ed.). Belmont, CA: Wadsworth.

Koh, H. K. (2002). Accomplishments of the Massachusetts Tobacco Control Program. *Tobacco Control, 11*(Suppl. 2), ii1–ii3.

Koopman, J. S., & Lynch, J. W. (1999). Individual causal models and population systems models in epidemiology. *American Journal of Public Health, 89,* 1170–1175.

Kreps, G. L., & Kunimoto, E. N. (1994). *Effective communication in multicultural health care settings.* Thousand Oaks, CA: Sage.

Kreuter, M., Farrell, D., Olevitch, L., & Brennan, L. (2000). *Tailored health messages: Customizing communication with computer technology.* Mahwah, NJ: Erlbaum.

Kroll, B., & Vann, R. J. (1981). *Exploring speaking-writing relationships: Connections and contrasts.* Urbana, IL: National Council for Teachers of English.

Kuruvilla, S., Dzenowagis, J., Pleasant, A., Dwivedi, R., Murthy, N., Samuel, R., & Scholtz, M. (2004). Digital bridges need concrete foundations: Lessons from the Health InterNetwork India. *BMJ, 328,* 1193–1196.

Labov, W. (1972). *Language in the inner city.* University Park: University of Pennsylvania Press.

Labov, W. (1994). *Principles of linguistic change.* Cambridge, MA: Blackwell.

LaForce, F. M., & Wussow, J. (2001). *Chronic illness in America: Overcoming barriers to building systems of care.* Center for Health Care Strategies, Consumer Action Series. July 2001. Retrieved Feb. 22, 2002, from http://www.chcs.org/publications/pdf/cas/bhschronicillness.pdf.

Lakoff, G. (2004). *Don't think of an elephant!* White River Junction, VT: Chelsea Green Publishing.

Lakoff, G., & Johnson, M. (1979). *Metaphors we live by.* Chicago: University of Chicago Press.

Lasker, R. D., & Weiss, E. S. (2003). Broadening participation in community problem solving: A multidisciplinary model to support collaborative practice and research. *Journal of Urban Health, 80*(1), 14–47.

Latour, B. (1987). *Science in action: How to follow scientists and engineers through society.* Cambridge, MA: Harvard University Press.

Laugksch, R. C. (2000). Scientific literacy: A conceptual overview. *Science Education, 84*(1), 71–94.

LaVeist, T. A. (Ed.). (2002). *Race, ethnicity, and health.* San Francisco: Jossey-Bass.

LeCompte, M. D., & Schensul, J. J. (1999a). *Analyzing and interpreting ethnographic data.* Walnut Creek, CA: Altamira Press.

LeCompte, M. D., & Schensul, J. J. (1999b). *Designing and conducting ethnographic research.* Walnut Creek, CA: Altamira Press.

Levy, D. T., & Friend, K. (2000). Gauging the effects of mass media policies: What do we need to know? *Journal of Public Health Management and Practice, 6*(3), 95–106.

Libby, R. T. (1995). *Eco-wars.* New York: Columbia University Press.

Lofland, J., & Lofland, L. H. (1995). *Analyzing social settings: Guide to qualitative observation and analysis* (3rd ed.). Belmont, CA: Wadsworth.

Long Island Breast Cancer Action Coalition (1in9). (n.d.). *1in9.org* [Web site]. Retrieved Jan. 30, 2004, from http://www.1in9.org.

Louis, M. R., & Sutton, R. I. (1991). Switching cognitive gears: From habits of mind to active thinking. *Human Relations, 44,* 55–76.

Luria, A. (1976). *Cognitive development: Its cultural and social foundations.* Cambridge, England: Cambridge University Press.

Mackay, J., & Eriksen, M. (2002). *The tobacco atlas* [Web site]. World Health Organization. Retrieved Mar. 23, 2003, from http://www5.who.int/tobacco/page.cfm?sid=84.

Maibach, E., & Parrott, R. L. (Eds.). (1995). *Designing health messages: Approaches from communication theory and public health practice*. Thousand Oaks, CA: Sage.

Mandler, J. M., & Johnson, N. S. (1977). Remembrance of things parsed: Story structure and recall. *Cognitive Psychology, 9*(1), 111–151.

March of Dimes. (2003). *Welcome to Peristats*. Retrieved Sept. 1, 2005, from http://www.marchofdimes.com/peristats/.

Marks, J. (2002). Folk heredity. In J. M. Fish (Ed.), *Race and intelligence: Separating science from myth* (pp. 95–112). Mahwah, NJ: Erlbaum.

McGee, J. (1999). *Writing and designing print materials for beneficiaries: A guide for state Medicaid agencies*. Baltimore, MD: Health Care Financing Administration, Center for Medicaid and State Operations.

McGuire, W. J. (1989). Theoretical foundations of campaigns. In C. K. Atkin (Ed.), *Public communication campaigns* (pp. 43–65). Thousand Oaks, CA: Sage.

McIntosh, J., & Blalock, S. J., (2005). Effects of media coverage of Women's Health Initiative study on attitudes and behavior of women receiving hormone replacement therapy. *American Journal of Health-System Pharmacy, 62*(1), 69–74.

McKenzie-Mohr, D., & Smith, W. (1999). *Fostering sustainable behavior: An introduction to community-based social marketing*. Gabriola Island, BC: New Society Publishers.

McLuhan, M. (1964). *Understanding the media: The extensions of man*. New York: McGraw-Hill.

McTaggart, R. (1997). Guiding principles for participatory action research. In R. McTaggart (Ed.), *Participatory action research: International contexts and consequences*. Albany: State University of New York Press.

Means, R. K. (1962). *A history of health education in the United States*. Philadelphia: Lea & Febiger.

Miller, J. D., & Kimmel, L. G. (2001). *Biomedical communications: Purposes, audiences, and strategies*. Orlando, FL: Academic Press.

Mintzes, B. (2002). Direct to consumer advertising is medicalising normal human experience. *BMJ, 324*, 908–909.

Morgan, D. L. (1993). *Successful focus groups: Advancing the state of the art*. Thousand Oaks, CA: Sage.

Mukherjee, A., & Vasanta, D. (Eds.). (2002). *Practice and research in literacy*. New Delhi, India: Sage India.

Muntaner, C., Lynch, J. L., & Smith, G. D. (2003). Social capital and the third way in public health. In R. Hofrichter (Ed.), *Health and social justice: Politics, ideology, and inequity in the distribution of disease*. San Francisco: Jossey-Bass.

Muro, A. (n.d.). *What is health literacy?* [Online article]. Boston: World Education. Retrieved Feb. 19, 2004, from http://www.worlded.org/us/health/lincs/muro.htm.

National Association of Attorney Generals. (n.d.). *Tobacco settlement agreement at a glance* [Web site]. Washington, DC: Author. Retrieved Dec. 10, 2003, from http://www.naag.org/issues/tobacco/msa_at_a_glance.php.

National Cancer Institute. (1994). *Clear and simple: Developing effective print materials for low-literate readers.* (NIH Publication No. 95–3594). Bethesda, MD: Author.

National Cancer Institute. (1999). *Smoking and tobacco control* (Tech. Rep.). Bethesda, MD: U.S. Department of Health and Human Services, National Institutes of Health, National Cancer Institute.

National Center for Chronic Disease Prevention and Health Promotion. (2001). *Statistics diabetes surveillance system preventive care practices: Prevalence of preventive care practices per 100 adults with diabetes, 42 states, 2001* [Web site]. Department of Health and Human Services, Centers for Disease Control and Prevention. Retrieved Aug. 15, 2003, from http://www.cdc.gov.

National Center for Health Statistics. (2001). *Infant mortality fact sheet.* Retrieved Sept. 1, 2005, from http://www.cdc.gov/omh/AMH/factsheets/infant.htm.

National Center for Health Statistics. (2004). *Health, United States* [Electronic version]. Retrieved July, 22, 2005, from http://www.cdc.gov/nchs/hus.htm.

National Center for the Study of Adult Learning and Literacy. (n.d.). [Web site]. Retrieved Feb. 16, 2004, from http://www.gse.harvard.edu/~ncsall/.

National Diabetes Information Clearinghouse. (2002). *Diabetes in American Indians and Alaska Natives* (Publication No. 02–4567). Washington, DC: National Institutes of Health.

National Foundation for Infantile Paralysis. (1947). *Facts and figures about infantile paralysis.* New York: Author.

National Foundation for Infantile Paralysis. (1952). *Polio pledge.* New York: Author.

National Foundation for Infantile Paralysis. (1954, June 1). *Press release.* New York: Author.

National Foundation for Infantile Paralysis. (1955, Jan. 31). *Bulletin for schools: Teachers' guide about the possibility of polio vaccinations.* New York: Author.

National Foundation for Infantile Paralysis. (1958a). *Brief history of National Foundation for Infantile Paralysis: Vaccination program to prevent paralytic polio.* New York: Author.

National Foundation for Infantile Paralysis. (1958b). *Sample radio announcements*. New York: Author.

National Foundation for Infantile Paralysis. (n.d.). *Annual numbers of cases of infantile paralysis reported and case rate per 100,000 population, by state, 1947–51*. New York: Author.

National Institute of Diabetes and Digestive and Kidney Diseases. (2003). *National diabetes statistics fact sheet: General information and national estimates on diabetes in the United States, 2003* [Electronic version]. U.S. Department of Health and Human Services, National Institutes of Health. Retrieved Feb. 2, 2004, from http://www.diabetes.niddk.nih.gov.

National Institute of Diabetes and Digestive and Kidney Diseases. (n.d.). *The Pima Indians: Focus on prevention* [Electronic version]. National Institute of Diabetes and Digestive and Kidney Diseases. Retrieved Jan. 29, 2004, from http://diabetes.niddk.nih.gov/dm/pubs/ppima/focus/focus.htm.

National Institute of General Medical Sciences, Office of Communications and Public Liaison. (2001). *Genes and populations*. Bethesda, MD: U.S. Department of Health and Human Services.

National Science Board. (2002, 2003, 2004). *Science and engineering indicators— 2002 and 2003*. Arlington, VA: National Science Foundation [Electronic version]. Retrieved Feb. 18, 2004, from http://www.nsf.gov/sbe/srs/seind93/chap7/doc/7d1a93.htm.

National Telecommunications and Information Administration. (2004). *A nation online: Entering the broadband age*. Retrieved July 22, 2005, from http://www.ntia.doc.gov/reports/anol/NationOnlineBroadband04.htm.

National Tuberculosis Association. (1945). *The story of TB and the NTA* (Pamphlet). Atlantic City, NJ: Author.

Nelkin, D. (1987). *Selling science: How the press covers science and technology*. New York: Freeman.

Neuberger, J. (2000). The educated patient: New challenges for the medical profession. *Journal of Internal Medicine, 247*, 6–10.

New York City Office of Emergency Management. (n.d.). *Utility disruption*. Retrieved Sept. 10, 2005, from http://www.nyc.gov/html/oem/html/readynewyork/hazard_utilities.html.

Nielsen-Bohlman, L., Panzer, A. M., & Kindig, D. A. (Eds.). (2004). *Health literacy: A prescription to end confusion*. Washington, DC: Institute of Medicine of the National Academies. Retrieved Feb. 1, 2005, from http://www.iom.edu/report.asp?id=19723.

Nutbeam, D. (1998). Evaluating health promotion—progress, problems and solutions. *Health Promotion International, 13*(1), 27–44.

Nutbeam, D. (1999). Literacies across the lifespan: Health literacy. *Literacy and Numeracy Studies, 9*(2), 47–55.

Nutbeam, D. (2000). Health literacy as a public health goal: A challenge for contemporary health education and communication strategies into the 21st century. *Health Promotion International, 15*(3), 259–267.

Nutbeam, D., & Kickbusch, I. (2000). Advancing health literacy: A global challenge for the 21st century. *Health Promotion International, 15*(3), 183–184.

O'Connor, F., Parker, E., & Oldenburg, B. (2000). Health promotion workforce development in Australia: Findings of a national study. *Health Promotion Journal of Australia, 10*(2), 140–147.

Olson, D. R. (1977). From utterance to text: The bias of language in speech and writing. *Harvard Educational Review, 47*, 257–281.

Olson, D. R. (Ed.). (1980). *The social foundations of language and thought: Essays in honor of Jerome S. Bruner.* New York: Norton.

Olson, D. R. (1994). *The world on paper.* Cambridge, England: Cambridge University Press.

Olson, D. R., & Torrance, N. (Eds.). (2001). *The making of literate societies.* Cambridge, MA: Blackwell.

Ong, L.M.L., de Haes, J., Hoos, A. M., & Lammes, F. B. (1995). Doctor-patient communication: A review of the literature. *Social Science Medicine, 40*(7), 903–918.

Orasanu, J. (Ed.). (1986). *Reading comprehension: From research to practice.* Mahwah, NJ: Erlbaum.

PACT Nepal. (n.d.). *Women's Empowerment Project* [Online press release]. Retrieved Feb. 8, 2004, from http://www.microcreditsummit.org/press/ PACT.htm.

Pardo, R., & Calvo, F. (2002). Attitudes toward science among the European public: A methodological analysis. *Public Understanding of Science, 11*, 155–195.

Park, P. (1993). What is participatory research? A theoretical and methodological perspective. In P. Park, J. Gaventa, T. Heaney, T. Jackson, J. Merrifield, B. D. Horton, D. E. Comstock, R. Fox, M. Brydon-Miker, M. B. Castellano, & P. Maguire (Eds.), *Voices of change: Participatory research in the United States and Canada* (pp. 1–19). Westport, CT: Bergin and Garvey.

Parker, R. M., Baker, D. W., Williams, M. V., & Nurss, J. R. (1995). The test of functional health literacy in adults: A new instrument for measuring patients' literacy skills. *Journal of General Internal Medicine, 10*(10), 537–541.

Partnership for Clear Health Communication (AskMe3). (2003). *Ask Me 3* [Web site]. Retrieved Feb. 9, 2004, from http://www.askme3.org.

Paterson, R. G. (1950). *Foundations of community health education.* New York: McGraw-Hill.

Patton, M. Q. (2003). *Qualitative research and evaluation methods* (3rd ed.). Thousand Oaks, CA: Sage.

Perkins, E. R., Simnett, I., & Wright, L. (Eds.). (1999). *Evidence-based health promotion.* West Sussex, England: Wiley.

Perkins, J. E. (1952). *You and tuberculosis* (1st ed.). New York: Knopf.

Pew Internet and American Life Project. (2005). *Health information online.* Retrieved July 22, 2005, from http://207.21.232.103/PPF/r/156/ report_display.asp.

Pew Research Center for the People and the Press. (2001a). *Public's news habits little changed by September 11* [Web site]. Washington, DC: Author. Retrieved Mar. 5, 2003, from http://people-press.org/reports/display. php3?PageID=613.

Pew Research Center for the People and the Press. (2001b). *No rise in fears or reported depression: Public remains steady in face of anthrax scare.* Washington, DC: Author.

Philip Morris USA. (n.d.). *Health issues: Second hand smoke* [Web site]. Retrieved Sept. 9, 2005, from http://www.philipmorrisusa.com/en/health_issues/ secondhand_smoke.asp.

Phillipov, G., & Phillips, P. J. (2003). Frequency of health-related search terms on the internet. *Journal of the American Medical Association, 290*(17), 2258–2259.

Pleasant, A., Kuruvilla, S., Zarcadoolas, C., Shanahan, J., & Lewenstein, B. (2003). *A framework for assessing public engagement with health research.* Geneva: World Health Organization. Retrieved Sept. 1, 2005, from http://www.aesop.rutgers.edu/~cils/pleasant_etal_who.pdf.

Posovac, H. D., Posovac, S. S., & Posovac, E. J. (1998). Exposure to media images of female attractiveness and concern with body weight among young women. *Sex Roles, 38*(3-4), 187–201.

Powers, R. (1988). Emergency department patient literacy and the readability of patient-directed materials. *Annals of Emergency Medicine, 17,* 124/135– 126/137.

PRAMS Working Group. (1997, Sept. 24). Prevalence of selected maternal and infant characteristics, Pregnancy Risk Assessment Monitoring System (PRAMS). *MMWR,* 1–37.

Preidt, R. (2005, July, 7). Preemie babies bring primo pricetags: Hospital bills now top $200,000 for tiniest newborns [Electronic version]. *HealthDay,*

July 7, 2005. Retrieved Sept. 1, 2005, from http://www.healthday.com/view.cfm?id=526559.

Price, E.L.G. (1952). *Pennsylvania pioneers against tuberculosis*. New York: National Tuberculosis Association.

Price, V., & Hsu, M. L. (1992). Public opinion about AIDS policies: The role of misinformation and attitudes toward homosexuals. *Public Opinion Quarterly, 56*(1), 29–52.

Prochaska, J. O., & DiClemente, C. C. (1983). Stages and processes of self-change of smoking: Toward an integrative model of change. *Journal of Consulting and Clinical Psychology, 51,* 390–395.

Prochaska, J. O., DiClemente, C. C., & Norcross, J. (1992). In search of how people change: Application to addictive behaviors. *American Psychologist, 47,* 1102–1114.

Propp, V. (1968). *Morphology of the folktale* (L. Scott, Trans., 2nd ed.). Austin: University of Texas Press.

Putnam, R. D. (1995). Tuning in, tuning out: The strange disappearance of social capital in America. *Political Science and Politics, 28*(4), 664–683.

Putnam, R. D. (2000). *Bowling alone: The collapse and revival of American community*. New York: Simon & Schuster.

Ragin, C. C. (1994). *Constructing social research*. Thousand Oaks, CA: Pine Forge Press.

Rao, S. D., & Rao, V.B.S. (2002). Evaluation of total literacy campaigns: The Andhra Pradesh experience. In D. Vasanta (Ed.), *Practice and research in literacy*. New Delhi, India: Sage India.

Ratzan, S. C. (2001). Health literacy: Communication for the public good. *Health Promotion International, 16*(2), 207–214.

Reagan, P. B., & Salsberry, P. J. (2005, May). Race and ethnic differences in determinants of preterm birth: Broadening the social context. *Social Science and Medicine, 60*(10), 2217–2228.

A revolution at 50: Kirk Bloodsworth. (2003, Feb. 25). *New York Times*, p. F5.

Risk, A., & Dzenowagis, J. (2001). Review of Internet health information quality initiatives. *Journal of Medical Internet Research, 3*(4), e28.

Robbins, H. (2002). Adult smoking intervention programmes in Massachusetts: A comprehensive approach with promising results. *Tobacco Control, 11*(Suppl. 2), ii4–ii7.

Robideaux, Y. D., Moore, K., Avery, C., Muneta, B., Knight, M., & Buchwald, D. (2000). Diabetes education materials: Recommendations of tribal leaders, Indian health professionals, and American Indian community members. *Diabetes Educator, 26*(2), 290–294.

Rogers, E. M., Ratzan, S. C., & Payne, J. G. (2001). Health literacy: A nonissue in the 2000 presidential election. *American Behavioral Scientist, 44*(12), 2172–2195.

Root, J., & Stableford, S. (1998). *Write it easy-to-read: A guide to creating plain English materials*. Biddeford, ME: Health Literacy Center, University of New England.

Root, J., & Stableford, S. (1999). Easy-to-read consumer communications: A missing link in Medicaid managed care. *Journal of Health Politics, Policy and Law, 24*(1), 1–26.

Rosenthal, M. B., Berndt, E. R., Donohue, J. M., Frank, R. G., & Epstein, A. M. (2002). Promotion of prescription drugs to consumers. *New England Journal of Medicine, 346*, 498–505.

Roter, D. L. (1984). Patient question asking in physician-patient interaction. *Health Psychology, 3*(5), 395–409.

Roter, D. L., & Hall, J. A. (1989). Studies of doctor-patient interaction. *Annual Review of Public Health, 10*, 163–180.

Roter, D. L., & Hall, J. A. (1992). *Doctors talking to patients/patients talking to doctors: Improving communication in medical visits*. Westport, CT: Auburn House.

Roussos, S. T., & Fawcett, S. B. (2000). A review of collaborative partnerships as a strategy for improving community health. *Annual Review of Public Health, 21*, 369–402.

Rudd, R. E. (2002). A maturing partnership. *Focus on Basics, 5*(c), 1–8.

Rudd, R. E., & Kirsch, I. (2003, Nov. 15). *Health literacy: Empowering disadvantaged populations*. Paper presented at the American Public Health Association Annual Meeting, San Francisco.

Rudd, R. E., Zacharia, C., & Daube, K. (1998). *Integrating health and literacy: Adult educators' experiences*. Boston: NCSALL/World Education.

Schank, R. C., & Abelson, R. P. (1977). *Scripts, plans, goals, and understanding: An inquiry into human knowledge structures*. Mahwah, NJ: Erlbaum.

Schillinger, D., Grumbach, K., Piette, J., Wang, F., Osmond, D., Daher, C., Palacios, J., Sullivan, G. D., & Bindman, A. B. (2002). Association of health literacy with diabetes outcomes. *Journal of the American Medical Association, 288*, 475–482.

Schwartzberg, J. G., VanGeest, J. B., & Wang, C. C. (Eds.). (2005). *Understanding health literacy: Implications for medicine and public health*. Chicago: AMA Press.

Scribner, S., & Cole, M. (1981). *The psychology of literacy*. Cambridge, MA: Harvard University Press.

Seale, C. (2002). *Media and health*. Thousand Oaks, CA: Sage.

Searle, J. R. (1969). *Speech acts: An essay in the philosophy of language*. Cambridge, England: Cambridge University Press.

Searle, J. R. (1993). Metaphor. In A. Ortony (Ed.), *Metaphor and thought* (2nd ed., pp. 83–111). Cambridge, England: Cambridge University Press.

Sen, A. (1999). *Development as freedom*. New York: Oxford University Press.

Shanahan, J., & Morgan, M. (1999). *Television and its viewers: Cultivation theory and research*. Cambridge, England: Cambridge University Press.

Shapiro, M. C., Najman, J. M., Chang, A., Keeping, J. D., Morrison, J., & Western, J. S. (1983). Information control and the exercise of power in the obstetrical encounter. *Social Science Medicine, 17*(3), 139–146.

Shilts, R. (1988). *And the band played on*. New York: Penguin.

Shryock, R. H., & Welch, W. H. (1957). *National Tuberculosis Association, 1904–1954*. New York: National Tuberculosis Association.

Shute, N. (2002, January 28). America's doctor. Portrait: Anthony Fauci. *U.S. News & World Report*, p. 32.

Signorelli, N. (1990). Television and health: Image and impact. In C. Atkin & L. Wallack (Eds.), *Mass communication and public health: Complexities and conflicts* (pp. 96–113). Thousand Oaks, CA: Sage.

Singer, E., Rogers, T. F., & Glassman, M. B. (1988). Public opinion about AIDS before and after the 1988 U.S. government public information campaign. *Public Opinion Quarterly, 55*(2), 161–279.

Singhal, A., & Rogers, E. M. (2003). *Combating AIDS: Community strategies in action*. Thousand Oaks, CA: Sage.

Slovic, P. (1987). Perception of risk. *Science, 236*(4799), 280–285.

Southern Newspaper Association. (2005). *Hurricane update*. Retrieved Sept. 10, 2005, from http://www.snpa.org/.

Starr, P. (1982). *The social transformation of American medicine*. New York: Basic Books.

Stice, E., & Shaw, H. E. (1994). Adverse effects of the media portrayed thin-ideal on women and linkages to bulimic symptomatology. *Journal of Social and Clinical Psychology, 13*(3), 288–308.

Stock, B. (1983). *The implications of literacy: Written language and models of interpretation in the eleventh and twelfth centuries*. Princeton, NJ: Princeton University Press.

Street, B. (Ed.). (1993a). *Cross-cultural approaches to literacy*. Cambridge, England: Cambridge University Press.

Street, B. (1993b). *Literacy in theory and practice*. Cambridge, England: Cambridge University Press.

Stubbs, M. (1983). *Discourse analysis: The sociolinguistic analysis of natural language*. Chicago and Oxford: University of Chicago Press and Blackwell.

Tannen, D. (Ed.). (1982). *Spoken and written language: Exploring orality and literacy*. Norwood, NJ: Ablex.

Tomes, N. (2000). The making of a germ panic, then and now. *American Journal of Public Health, 90*(2), 191–198.

Tresserras, R., Canela, J., Alvarez, J., Sentis, J., & Salleras, L. (1992). Infant mortality, per capita income and adult illiteracy: An ecological approach. *American Journal of Public Health, 82*(3), 435–438.

UCLA study shows Head Start training lowers Medicaid costs [Press release]. (2004, Apr. 15). Retrieved Apr. 21, 2006, from http://www.anderson.ucla.edu/x1628.xml.

Ulin, P. R., Robinson, E. T., & Tolley, E. E. (2005). *Qualitative methods in public health: A field guide for applied research*. San Francisco: Jossey-Bass.

United Health Foundation (UHF). (2003). *Get smart: Know when antibiotics work*. Retrieved Sept. 10, 2005, from http://www.unitedhealthfoundation.org/anti.html.

United Nations Educational Scientific and Cultural Organization (UNESCO). (2003). *Literacy as freedom: A UNESCO roundtable* [Electronic version]. Paris: Literacy and Non-Formal Education Section, Division of Basic Education, UNESCO. Retrieved Sept. 10, 2005, from http://unesdoc.unesco.org/images/0013/001318/131823e.pdf.

United Nations Educational Scientific and Cultural Organization. (2005). *Education for all: Literacy for life*. Paris: Author. Retrieved Feb. 13, 2006, from http://unesdoc.unesco.org/images/0014/001416/141639e.pdf.

U.S. Census Bureau. (2003). *Language use and English-speaking ability*. Washington, DC: Author.

U.S. Department of Agriculture. (2005a). *Statement by Dr. John Clifford regarding further analysis of BSE inconclusive test results, June 10, 2005* [Electronic version]. Press release no. 0206.05. Retrieved Sept. 1, 2005, from http://www.usda.gov/wps/portal/!ut/p/_s.7_0_A/7_0_1OB?contentidonly=true&contentid=2005/06/0206.xml.

U.S. Department of Agriculture. (2005b). *Steps to a healthier you* [Web site]. Retrieved Sept. 1, 2005, from http://www.mypyramid.gov/.

U.S. Department of Health and Human Services. (1986). *The health consequences of involuntary smoking*. Rockville, MD: U.S. Department of Health and Human Services Public Health Service, Centers for Disease Control, Center for Health Promotion and Education, Office on Smoking and Health.

U.S. Department of Health and Human Services. (2000). *Healthy people 2010: National health promotion and disease prevention objectives*: Washington, DC: U.S. Department of Health and Human Services. Retrieved June 10, 2005, from http://www.healthy.gov/healthypeople.

U.S. Department of Health and Human Services. (2003). The power of prevention: Steps to a healthier U.S. program and policy perspective. Retrieved Jan. 25, 2006, from http://www.healthierus.gov/steps/summit/prevportfolio/power/index.html#we.

U.S. Department of Health and Human Services, Health Resources and Services Administration. (2004). The power of partnership: Meeting today's MCH challenges through partnerships, MCH training program. *Cultural and Linguistic Competency in Curricula and Training Workgroup*, October 5–6, 2004. Retrieved Sept. 1, 2005, from http://mchb.hrsa.gov/training/documents/event_resources/4_Cultural__Linguistic_Competencies.htm.

U.S. Food and Drug Administration. (2003). *Easy-to-read publications*. Retrieved Dec. 3, 2003, from http://www.fda.gov/opacom/lowlit/7lowlit.html.

U.S. Government Accountability Office. (2004, May 19). Department of Health and Human Services, Centers for Medicare & Medicaid Services [Video news releases, B-302710]. May 19, 2004. Retrieved July 20, 2005, from http://www.gao.gov/decisions/appro/302710.htm.

U.S. National Science Board. (2004). *Science and engineering indicators 2004*. Arlington, VA: Author. Retrieved Jan. 8, 2006, from http://www.nsf.gov/statistics/seind04.

U.S. Postal Service. (2001). *Security of the mail: Postcard* [Web site]. Author. Retrieved Apr. 2, 2002, from http://www.usps.gov/news/2001/press/mailsecurity/postcard.htm.

Valdiserri, R. O. (2002). HIV/AIDS stigma: An impediment to public health. *American Journal of Public Health, 92*(3), 341–342.

Valdiserri, R. O. (Ed.). (2003). *Dawning answers: How the HIV/AIDS epidemic has helped to strengthen public health*. New York: Oxford University Press.

van Dijk, T. (1977). *Text and context: Explorations in the semantics and pragmatics of discourse*. White Plains, NY: Longman.

Vygotsky, L. S. (1962). *Thought and language*. Cambridge, MA: MIT Press.

Wade, N. (2000, June 27). Reading the book of life: The overview; genetic code of life is cracked by scientists. *New York Times*, p. A1.

Wallack, L. (1990). Mass media and health promotion: Promise, problem, and challenge. In C. Atkin & L. Wallack (Eds.), *Mass communication and public health: Complexities and conflicts* (pp. 13–40). Thousand Oaks, CA: Sage.

Walter, P. (1999). Defining literacy and its consequences in the developing world. *International Journal of Lifelong Education, 18*(1), 31–48.

Watson, J. D. (1990). The human genome project: Past, present, and future. *Science, 248*(4951), 44–48.

Webb, D. (1999). Current approaches to gathering evidence. In E. R. Perkins, I. Simnett, & L. Wright (Eds.), *Evidence-based health promotion* (pp. 34–46). Hoboken, NJ: Wiley.

Weller, S. C., Baer, R. D., Pachter, L. M., Trotter, R. T., Glazer, M., Garcia, G.D.A., Javier, E., & Klein, R. E. (1999). Latino beliefs about diabetes. *Diabetes Care, 22*(5), 722–727.

Wilkinson, R. G. (1996). *Unhealthy societies: The afflictions of inequality.* New York: Routledge.

Williams, M. V., Baker, D. W., Parker, R. M., & Nurss, J. R. (1998). Relationship of functional health literacy to patient's knowledge of their chronic disease: A study of patients with hypertension or diabetes. *Archives of Internal Medicine, 158*, 166–172.

Williams, M., Parker, R., Baker, D., Parikh, K., Coates, W., & Nurss, J. (1995). Inadequate functional health literacy among patients at two public health hospitals. *Journal of the American Medical Association, 2714*, 1677–1682.

Wilson, B.D.M., & Miller, R. L. (2003). Examining strategies for culturally grounded HIV prevention: A review. *AIDS Education and Prevention, 15*(2), 184–202.

Winfrey, O. (2006, Jan. 24). Bird flu: The untold story (Interview with Dr. Michael Osterholm). *Oprah Winfrey Show.* Retrieved Mar. 7, 2006, from http://www2.oprah.com/tows/pastshows/200601/tows_past_20060124.jhtml.

Winterbottom, C., Liska, D., & Obermaier, K. M. (1995). *State-level databook of health care access and financing* (2nd ed.). Washington, DC: Urban Institute.

Wolitski, R. J., Valdiserri, R. O., Denning, P., & Levine, W. (2001). Are we headed for a resurgence of the HIV epidemic among men who have sex with men? *American Journal of Public Health, 91*(6), 883–888.

Woods, D. (1991). America responds to AIDS: Its content, development, process, and outcome. *Public Health Reports, 106*(6), 616–622.

World Bank. (1999). "Social capital." *PovertyNet.* Retrieved Jan. 7, 2006, from http://web.worldbank.org/WBSITE/EXTERNAL/TOPICS/EXTSOCIALDEVELOPMENT/EXTTSOCIALCAPITAL/0,,menuPK:401021~pagePK:149018~piPK:149093~theSitePK:401015,00.html.

World Bank. (2002). *Social capital and development* [Web site]. World Bank's Social Capital Team, Social Development Department. Retrieved Mar. 12, 2003, from http://www.iris.umd.edu/socat/concept.htm.

World Education. (2004). *World education* [Web site]. Retrieved Feb. 15, 2004, from www.worlded.org

World Health Organization. (1986). *Ottawa Charter for Health Promotion* [Web site]. Copenhagen: Author. Retrieved Feb. 16, 2004, from http://www.who.dk/AboutWHO/Policy/20010827_2.

World Health Organization. (1998). *Health promotion glossary* [Online]. Division of Health Promotion, Education and Communications, Health Education and Health Promotion Unit. Retrieved Feb. 15, 2004, from http://www.who.int/hpr/NPH/docs/hp_glossary_en.pdf.

World Health Organization, United Nations Population Fund, United Nations Children's Fund, & World Bank. (1999). *Factors underlying the medical causes: Reduction of maternal mortality* [Online report]. Retrieved Feb. 19, 2004, from http://www.who.int/reproductive-health/publications/reduction_of_maternal_mortality/reduction_maternal_mortality_chap2.htm.

Young, J. H. (1985). Patent medicines and the self-help syndrome. In R. L. Numbers (Ed.), *Sickness and health in America: Readings in the history of medicine and public health.* Madison: University of Wisconsin Press.

Young, J. H. (1988). Patent medicines: An element in southern distinctiveness? In J. H. Young (Ed.), *Disease and distinctiveness in the American South.* Knoxville: University of Tennessee Press.

Zarcadoolas, C., Ahern, D., & Blanco, M. (1997). *How to evaluate information from providers: Tools for non-mainstream populations* (Phase I Final Rep. No. 290-97-0002). Rockville, MD: Agency for Health Care Policy and Research/Small Business Innovation Research.

Zarcadoolas, C., & Blanco, M. (2000). Lost in translation: Each word accurate, yet . . . *Managed Care, 9*(8), 22A–22F.

Zarcadoolas, C., Blanco, M., Boyer, F., & Pleasant, A. (2002). Unweaving the web: An exploratory study of low-literate adults' navigation skills on the World Wide Web. *Journal of Health Communication, 7*(4), 309–324.

Zarcadoolas, C., Blanco, M., Lane, P., Rojas, M., Smith, H., & Boyer, J. (2004). *Simplifying Medicaid/SCHIP enrollment and retention forms.* Final Report submitted to DHHS/CMS, 2004.

Zarcadoolas, C., Pleasant, A., & Greer, D.S. (2005, June). Understanding health literacy: An expanded model. *Health Promotion International, 20,* 195–203.

Zarcadoolas, C., Timm, E., & Bibeault, L. (2001). Brownfields: A case study in partnering with residents to develop an easy-to-read print guide. *Journal of Environmental Health, 64*(1), 15–20.

Name Index

Subject Index